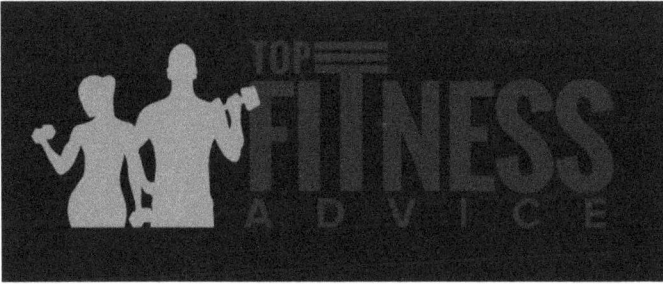

HEALTH

4th Edition

139 POWERFUL & Scientifically PROVEN Health Tips to Boost Your Health, Shed Pounds & Live Longer!

LINDA WESTWOOD

ink

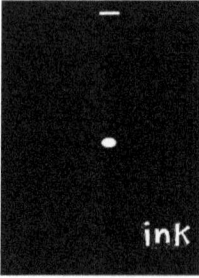

Disclaimer

This book provides wellness management information in an informative and educational manner only, with information that is general in nature and that is not specific to you, the reader. The contents of this book are intended to assist you and other readers in your personal wellness efforts. Consult your physician regarding the applicability of any information provided in this book to you.

Nothing in this book should be construed as personal advice or diagnosis, and must not be used in this manner. The information provided about conditions is general in nature. This information does not cover all possible uses, actions, precautions, side-effects, or interactions of medicines, or medical procedures. The information in this book should not be considered as complete and does not cover all diseases, ailments, physical conditions, or their treatment.

You should consult with your physician before beginning any exercise, weight loss, or health care program. This book should not be used in place of a call or visit to a competent health-care professional. You should consult a health care professional before adopting any of the suggestions in this book or before drawing inferences from it.

Any decision regarding treatment and medication for your condition should be made with the advice and consultation of a qualified health care professional. If you have, or suspect you have, a health-care problem, then you should immediately contact a qualified health care professional for treatment.

No Warranties: The author and publisher don't guarantee or warrant the quality, accuracy, completeness, timeliness, appropriateness or suitability of the information in this book, or of any product or services referenced in this book.

The information in this book is provided on an "as is" basis and the author and publisher make no representations or warranties of any kind with respect to this information. This book may contain inaccuracies, typographical errors, or other errors.

Table of Contents

Would you prefer to listen to my book, rather than read it?

Download the audiobook version for free!

If you go to the special link below and sign up to Audible as a new customer, you can get the audiobook version of my book completely free.

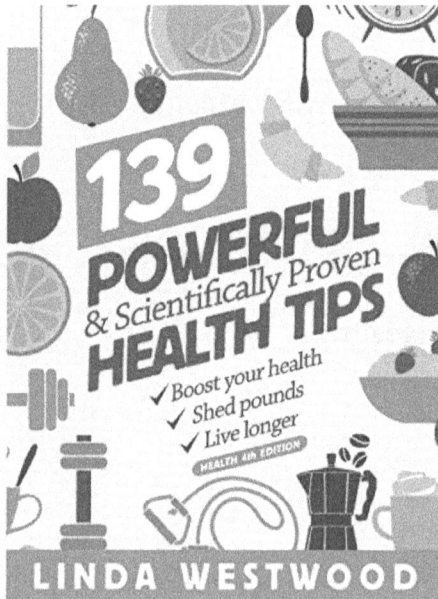

Go here to get your audiobook version for free:

TopFitnessAdvice.com/go/health139

Who is this book for?

This book is perfect if:

- You are looking to get a *strong* kick-start with your weight loss!

- You wish your fat would just fall off *effortlessly!*

- You are ready to BOOST health and FEEL GREAT all day, every day!

- Or you WANT a full body transformation that is tailored for women!

I am going to share with you the most effective way to slim down and get flat abs, a firm butt and lean legs!

I am also going to share with you some of the MOST EFFECTIVE, MOST POWERFUL, and EASIEST health tips that you can add into your life today, to quickly boost health, wellbeing and energy levels!

The best part about is that you are going to see amazing results and this will *TRANSFORM YOUR BODY IN A VERY SHORT TIME – days, not weeks*!

You can be a complete beginner or someone who is already healthy, it doesn't matter! If this sounds like it could help you, then keep reading...

What will this book teach you?

Inside, I will teach you one of the best ways to transform your body and health, especially your belly, butt and thighs, which will not only boost your weight loss, but also rejuvenate both your mind and body!

You will feel the healthiest you have ever felt – have the most energy you have ever had – and the fat will be melting *effortlessly!*

How?

Because you're going to be eating well, and following some of the most effective health tips that accelerate body transformation in a short period of time.

In this book, I give you the plan right in front of you that will change your life – all you have to do is follow it!

One of the most important things for you to realize when reading this book is that it *really does work!*

However...

For you to achieve *real success*, you HAVE to apply this to your life.

This is where most people fail – they read through the entire book but do nothing.

You MUST try your best to apply as you read through the book!

Introduction

Getting healthy and losing weight can be one of the greatest challenges any person goes through. This is especially the case for women whose bodies are biologically more likely to put on weight—especially in the belly, butt, and thighs.

Getting rid of those extra pounds means quitting bad habits and adopting good habits all while maintaining the physical and emotional strength to keep up with all of your other responsibilities in life.

If all you had to worry about in life was your weight, then it would be easy.

But if you're like most people, you have a million other things on your plate right now and it can seem nearly impossible to make weight loss a priority.

But it *is* possible!

You can make a weight loss plan that fits with your schedule and your abilities. This book is here to help you do that. It's not about major life changes, extreme diets, or brutal workouts.

It's about all the small changes you can make that will eventually add up to help you lose all that extra weight and get down to that dream figure!

Instead of trying (and failing) to find the time to work out for an hour every morning or prepare complex weight loss meals 3 times per day; you can slowly incorporate these changes to transform your life and lose the weight for good.

In this book, you'll get genius tips for losing weight and becoming healthier overall. Remember, losing weight isn't enough by itself, you also need to feel better each and every day. You need to be energized in the morning, and never feel bloated again!

These tips will work for anyone but they are especially designed to help women with that stubborn belly, butt, and thigh fat – as well as feeling better every day, and improving their overall health.

In addition to these tips, you'll get some bonuses – amazing workouts that target belly fat *and* workouts for the butt and thigh area!

With so many tips and workout options, your weight loss plan will never get dull and you'll be able to stay motivated to keep making the necessary changes to finally get rid of those stubborn pounds once and for all!

Discover Scientifically-Proven "Shortcuts" & "Hacks" to Lose Weight FASTER (With Very Little Effort)

For this month only, you can get Linda's best-selling & most popular book absolutely free – *Weight Loss Secrets You NEED to Know.*

Get Your FREE Copy Here:
TopFitnessAdvice.com/Bonus

Discover scientifically-proven tips to help you lose weight faster and easier than ever before. With this book, readers were able to improve their weight loss results and fitness levels. So, it's highly recommended that you get this book, especially while it's free!

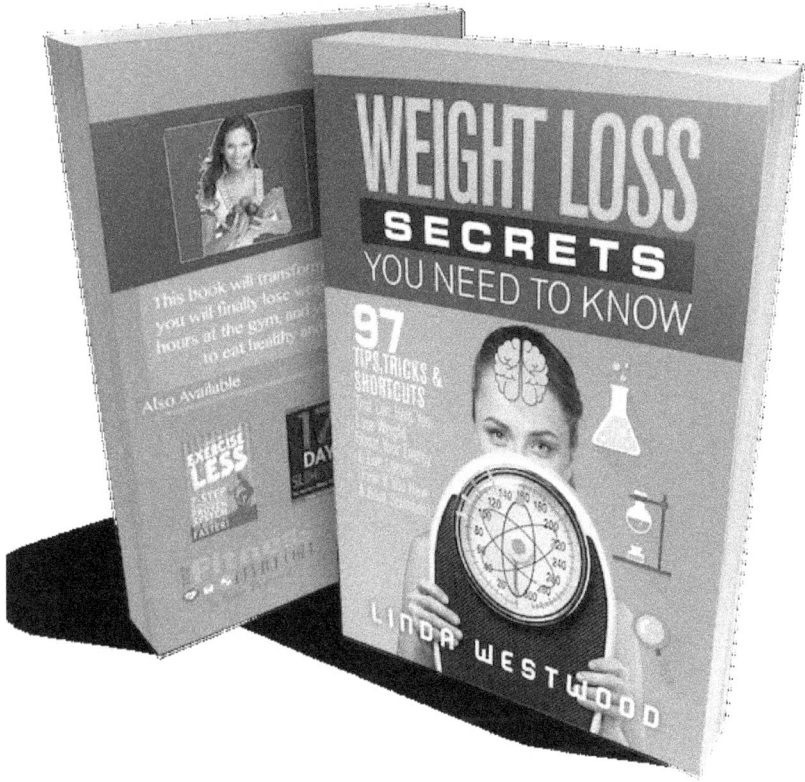

Get Your FREE Copy Here:

TopFitnessAdvice.com/Bonus

Top Tips to Get Rid of Belly Fat

This first section will focus on tips for burning off the extra fat that's been building up around your belly, while trimming down your waistline.

The tips focus on diet, exercise, and lifestyle changes that you can make.

As I said in the introduction, this book isn't about extreme diets or workouts.

It's about making simple changes to your lifestyle that you can maintain in the long run so that the pounds will melt away and stay gone for good.

The best way to make sure that you successfully turn these tips into full habits is to take it one step at a time.

Don't overwhelm yourself by trying to make all the changes at once.

Getting healthy and achieving permanent weight loss is a long journey.

If you want to do it right and make sure the weight stays off, you have to take your time and make sure you are really working on turning these into your new, healthy habits that replace the old unhealthy habits you used to have.

Health Tip #1 – Go for Variety Over Reps

A lot of people think of working out as doing the same thing over and over until your muscles are totally fatigued and screaming in pain.

But to make your exercise the most effective, you want to work smart, not hard.

Instead of doing 100 sit ups in one session, do 24 repetitions of 4 different workouts. This way, you target multiple muscle groups and strengthen different areas. The more muscles you target, the more fat you will burn.

This is because muscle burns up more calories (even when you are resting) than fat. Your body uses more calories to maintain muscles than it does to maintain fat.

So, while 100 sit-ups would certainly show some results, you're only targeting a limited range of muscles by doing just one move.

If you go for variety instead f maxing yourself out on one workout, you'll build more muscles in different areas all in a single workout session.

In the long run, this will lead to more fat loss and make it easier to keep the weight off for good.

Aside from the fact that variety helps your body lose more weight and keep the weight off, it also prevents injury. If you keep doing the same workout every day that only targets one specific group of muscles, you'll end up causing too much strain to those muscles.

You need to keep your workouts balanced so that all of your muscles are getting the exercise they need without any one muscle group getting worked to the point of exhaustion. This will help you avoid tearing muscles.

It will also prevent you from having uneven muscle development. Imagine a weight lifter who only lifts with the same arm every day.

Eventually, the weight lifter would have one bulky, muscular arm and one flabby, weak arm.

The same could happen with an imbalanced ab workout. Sit-ups target the muscles in the center of your abdomen. They don't do much for the muscles on your left or right side.

It's better to do a variety of workouts that each focus on different set of muscles in your abdomen to see the best results and make sure that your body is toned and evenly developed.

This is also the best way to make sure you don't get bored or burnt out on any single workout.

Health Tip #2 – Work Your Abs, Not Your Neck

If you're trying to build muscle and lose fat in your abdominal area, then you need to make sure the power is coming from your abs during the workout.

This may sound obvious but many people make the mistake of doing the workout wrong.

This is especially the case during sit-ups or crunches. Even if you start out by lifting with your abs, you often start to slack on your form as the muscles start to feel the burn.

Many people will start straining their neck to propel themselves upward in order to try and take some of the strain off of their stomach.

But this is counterproductive. The strain should be on your abs. That's the muscle group you want to work on when you're doing sit-ups or crunches.

Straining your neck isn't going to help you burn fat in the belly. Plus, it's going to put you at risk for causing serious damage to the muscles in your neck.

So, when you are doing your workouts, make sure that you pay attention to your form and movement throughout the exercise.

When doing sit ups, for example, you want the movement to be coming from the waist. Your lower back and abdomen should be doing all the work while your upper body is just following through.

Keep your mind focused on your core. Try to visualize the muscles that are working to accomplish the move and focus on using only those muscles for each repetition of the workout.

Go at a steady pace through each repetition. If you speed through them too quickly because you're just trying to get it over with, you'll have a harder time maintaining form.

So instead, slow it down and really focus on becoming aware of your body and the way each muscle is flexing and working together to complete a full repetition.

This doesn't mean you should go at a snail's pace and take breaks between repetitions. Instead, just focus on your form and your muscles and making sure that you are doing each repetition flawlessly. Don't worry about how quickly or slowly you finish a full set of repetitions.

As you get better, you'll be able to go at a faster speed but the speed is not important here. It's about the quality of each repetition, not how fast you can get through them all or how many you can do in a single minute.

You'll get more out of a workout session if you do fewer repetitions but do them all properly.

Health Tip #3 – Blast Ab Flab with Cardio

Belly fat builds up quickly but, unlike the fat that builds up in your butt and thighs, it also burns quickly.

When you start to maximize the number of calories you burn in a day, the first place your body is going to take fat from is your stomach.

This is where it will get the extra energy to fuel your increased physical activity.

So, if you're trying to burn belly fat, a good cardio routine is going to be essential. Cardio burns more calories per minute than strength training.

And those extra calories burned are primarily going to be taken from your belly since the fat stored in your butt and thighs are reserved for long-term use.

This doesn't mean you should only focus on cardio and totally skip any strength training. It just means you should include cardio as a regular part of your plan.

The ideal workout will be a combination of both so that you are maximizing calorie burn to get rid of that belly fat as soon as possible while also building muscle so that you can help ensure that your body will burn calories more efficiently in the long run.

One of the best parts of cardio is that there are so many options out there. If you can't stand running, you can try any of the other countless cardio activities. You could try cycling, swimming, hiking, dancing, or even a sport.

You just need to follow one simple guideline with any cardio activity that you choose: raise your heart rate above its normal resting rate for at least 20 consecutive minutes.

Your ideal range for maximum weight loss is 30 to 45 minutes but 20 minutes is the minimum threshold you need to reach.

As long as you are doing an activity that gets your blood pumping and your heart rate elevated for a minimum of 20 minutes, you are going to reap the fat-blasting rewards of a cardio workout.

Health Tip #4 – Short, Powerful Workouts WORK

You have probably gone most of your life hearing that in order for a workout to be the most effective, it has to be long, drawn out, and miserable.

For a long time, this is what people thought an effective workout looked like.

But luckily, scientific research has started to tell a different story. Decades of research has shown that our bodies get the maximum benefit with short but highly intense exercise rather than from endurance training.

This means that if you push your body to its limits for just a short time, you'll get more benefits than if you were to do a longer workout at a lower intensity.

Of course, the high intensity will wear you out but you can motivate yourself with the thought that you only need to maintain this intensity for a short time.

Anyone can survive the high intensity for just 10 short minutes. And 10 minutes is all you need if you push yourself as hard as you can for that time.

And once you have survived those 10 minutes, you can rest with the confidence of knowing that you have accomplished your weight loss goals for the day.

The other benefit of this method is that you can probably find 10 spare minutes in your schedule no matter how busy you are. Wake up 10 minutes earlier or go to bed 10 minutes later.

Take a 10-minute workout break at work instead of the coffee break. The workout will leave you feeling far more energized than any cup of coffee ever could.

Health Tip #5 – Know When to Rest

So far, we have been focused on how to maximize the fat-burning power of your workout. But working out is not the whole story. Taking the time to rest between workouts is just as important as the workout itself.

In general, it is recommended that you never workout more than 2 or 3 days in a row. That means you should have two rest days per week.

This is important even if you don't feel like you need a rest day. You might be feeling pumped and ready to go but your body, especially your muscles, need time to rest and repair themselves.

So even if you feel fine, don't push yourself too hard. For the last tip, we talked about how it's important to push yourself *to* your limit. But it's also important to make sure you don't push yourself *past* your limit.

Your rest days are the times when your body will have a chance to repair muscles and build them up so that they are stronger than they were before.

By giving your body this time to rest and repair, you will be able to push your limit further and further so that you can make your workouts progressively more intense.

In addition to schedule in regular rest days, it's important to listen to what your body is telling you. If you feel sore or in pain the day after a workout, take that day to rest.

This soreness is a message from your body telling you that it needs some time to build up those muscles and get you ready for the next workout.

If you push yourself to exercise even when your muscles are in pain, you'll end up causing yourself serious injury that could keep you from your workout for weeks or even months.

It's better to take a rest day every now and then as needed than to risk being bed ridden for months and losing all that progress you have made.

Health Tip #6 – Clean!

Household chores may not exactly scream "excitement" but they do provide you with a good chance to burn off some extra calories.

And since keeping the house clean is probably already a part of your busy schedule, you can feel good knowing that it is also helping you accomplish your weight loss goals. You're killing two birds with one stone: getting your house clean and shedding those extra pounds!

So, make the most of it. Don't find the lazy or easy way to clean. Really get down and start scrubbing, vacuuming, and scouring.

Vacuuming is an especially great activity for your belly. Make sure to bend from your waist rather than your shoulders as you push the vacuum across the floor to maximize the ab workout you're getting from this household chore.

Also, focus on tightening your tummy as you go through the motions to make it an even more powerful workout.

Burning calories isn't all about doing weight loss workouts. It's also about maximizing the calories you burn just from your daily activities.

Cleaning and organizing your home is one of the best non-workout ways to lose weight.

Focus on body awareness. Pay attention to the muscles that are being used to accomplish each chore and then try to maximize the workout in those muscles.

Tighten and flex them as you go through your normal chores.

Health Tip #7 – Increase Fiber Intake

Fiber is not only essential for your health, it's also essential for effective weight loss. Most Americans do not get nearly enough fiber in their diet. The recommended minimum is between 25 and 30 grams while most people are only eating around 15 grams!

Before we talk about how fiber will help you lose weight, let's just take a quick look at exactly what fiber does.

It is an essential tool for your digestive system. It's what helps your body break down food efficiently and absorb the nutrients. It helps keep things moving along smoothly through your system. If you feel constipated, gassy, or bloated, it's likely because you aren't eating enough fiber.

For those who don't eat enough on a regular basis, their digestive system gets backed up. This means they aren't able to break down and absorb nutrients as quickly. It also means they will get bloated and constipated. They may also feel fatigued or lack energy during the day.

The longer food stays stuck in your system undigested, the more problems it causes. Not only will it lead to weight gain, it will also lead to serious health problems.

For example, low fiber diets have been found to be a major factor in colon cancer and other cancers of the digestive system.

So, how does more fiber lead to more weight loss? It's quite simple. Getting enough fiber means your digestive system will start operating more efficiently.

You'll be able to break down food into usable nutrients and your body will be able to absorb them and send them to where they need to go. You'll feel less bloated and you'll retain less water since your digestive system will no longer be clogged up.

Before you start increasing your fiber intake, spend 2 or 3 days checking how much fiber you get in your current diet. If you suddenly increase your daily fiber intake from 15 up to 30 at once, you'll shock the system. It'll feel like your digestive system has suddenly gone into overdrive.

Instead, add more fiber gradually. Add 5 grams per week. After going the whole week eating 5 extra grams of fiber each day, you can add another 5 grams. Do this until you get to 30 grams per day.

The best foods for fiber include beans of all kinds, oatmeal, whole grain foods, and non-starchy fruits and vegetables like carrots, apples, or raspberries.

Health Tip #8 – Reduce Salt Intake

If you eat a high salt diet, your first step should be to cut your salt down to healthy levels. That doesn't mean eliminate it entirely. Your body does need some salt in order to function properly.

It just means get rid of the excess salt because too much salt can cause serious health problems and serious weight gain.

The main function of salt in your diet is to help your body retain water long enough that it can use it to hydrate itself. If you ate absolutely no salt, the water would just drain right through you without getting delivered to your blood stream and cells.

However, when we eat too much salt (and *most* of us eat too much salt), we end up retaining way more water than we actually need. The excess water leads to bloating and weight gain in the form of "water weight." This water weight sticks to your belly area.

By decreasing salt intake, you'll quickly shed this water weight, which could make a dramatic difference depending on how much salt you normally eat.

The recommended daily intake is 2,300 mg of salt per day. You're already getting about 1/3 of that if you eat a single fast food cheeseburger. And just because a food doesn't really taste salty doesn't mean it is low in salt.

If you get a soda to go along with that cheeseburger, you're consuming another 19 to 30 mg of salt!

If you eat a lot of processed foods, this is probably where most of your salt is coming from. Studies show that about 90% of Americans eat too much salt. And by "too much" I really mean too much.

As mentioned above, the recommended intake is 2,300 mg per day. But the average American eats about 3,500 per day. That's nearly double the amount recommended every single day. But only about 10% of that salt is actually coming from the salt you sprinkle on yourself. The other 90% is hidden in foods (especially foods you don't really expect to be high in salt).

When you buy foods that are ready made or processed (junk food, convenience food, etc.), you're buying a whole lot of extra, unnecessary salt.

So, check the labels on the food you buy and start eating more whole foods that don't need to have ingredient labels because they have no added ingredients. Fresh fruits, vegetables, meats, and dairy products are all naturally low in salt and naturally high in flavor.

If you switch to a diet of whole, unprocessed foods, you won't even need to watch your salt intake so closely because you can be confident in knowing that the only salt in your diet is the salt you added. And as you read earlier, the salt you actually add yourself only accounts for about 10% of the total amount.

If you are like 90% of Americans, then you only add about 350 mg of salt on your own. If you switch to a natural, no salt added, whole food diet, you could add *six times* the amount you currently do and still fall below the recommended 2,300 mg allowance.

All that is to say that reducing salt intake isn't even a challenge. It's just a matter of eating the right foods so that you aren't consuming so much hidden salt. Once you do that, you'll watch the pounds melt off without even needing to stress about salt.

Health Tip #9 – Eat Avocado

Some diets will caution against eating avocados because they are high in fat. But what these diets don't understand is that eating fat does not necessarily lead to fat. In fact, if you eat the right kind of fat, it actually helps you lose weight!

Avocados are packed with exactly the kind of fat you need to lose weight: unsaturated fat. Understanding the difference between good and bad fat is key to weight loss. Think of unsaturated fats as the unprocessed, raw fats. Because it's unsaturated, your body works harder to digest it.

This is also the fat that your body needs in order to absorb nutrients more effectively. Many of the nutrients you need are "fat soluble" which means they can only be broken down and absorbed if they are coated in unsaturated fats.

This is exactly why more and more studies are showing that taking vitamin supplements is not as effective as just eating healthy foods that naturally contain those vitamins. Your body can't break down a tablet full of vitamins unless those vitamins are diluted with either unsaturated fat or water (depending on which kind of vitamin we are talking about).

A single avocado contains 20 grams of unsaturated fat. This high content of good fats will not only help you absorb nutrients better, it will help you feel full and satisfied longer. Both of these facts will lead to weight loss.

So, whenever you find yourself with a serious craving for fatty foods, reach for an avocado (or another food with unsaturated fats). At the same time, avoid the other kinds of fat: saturated fats and Trans fats.

Trans fats are your biggest enemy if you're trying to lose weight and should be completely cut out of your diet. Saturated fats are safe as long as you keep them to a minimum.

Health Tip #10 – No More Soda

If you're a soda drinker, this is probably one of the leading causes of your weight gain. Soda is packed full of more sugar than you could possibly imagine. If you were to try to eat that quantity of sugar in a single sitting (just like you do when you drink a soda) you'd feel sick and probably never want to eat sugar again.

Diet soda isn't any better. The sugar substitutes that they use are just as bad for you—if not worse—than the sugar they are trying to replace. Studies have shown that diet sodas lead to at least as much weight gain as their sugary counterparts so you're not helping yourself just by switching to diet.

While most people mistakenly think that eating fatty foods leads to gaining fat on your body, the fact is that sugar is by far the biggest culprit in weight gain. Sugar wreaks havoc on your digestive system, your circulation, and your metabolism.

It puts a lot of pressure on your entire body by causing huge energy spikes followed by sudden crashes, meaning your body is constantly swinging from one extreme to the other without ever being able to achieve a balance.

Cutting out soda from your life entirely is one of the biggest favors you could do for your body. You'll start dropping pounds faster than you can keep track and you'll just feel better and healthier overall.

If you are dependent on your soda habit, you'll want to either cut down gradually over time or find someone who can support you in going cold turkey. Yes, it can be a legitimate addiction. Your body starts to expect and need that sugar to function.

At the same time that you kick your soda habit, make sure to increase the fiber and unsaturated fats in your diet. Both of these will help maintain your energy levels and alleviate the "withdrawal" symptoms you will feel from giving up soda.

The health and weight loss results you will see are totally worth the struggle of getting over your soda dependency.

Health Tip #11 – Cut Out Alcohol

Alcohol can also lead to a lot of weight gain. The "beer belly" is not a figure of speech. Alcohol messes up your metabolism by redirecting it from burning fat to burning alcohol.

This is because your body can't store alcohol so it burns it immediately which means that the entire time you are drinking as well as the time afterward when you are dealing with the hangover, your body is not burning any fat. It's just struggling to burn all that alcohol.

Getting "light" beer or low-calorie drinks isn't going to make a difference either. The problem isn't the calories. It's the alcohol itself.

It's ok to enjoy a glass now and then but if you overdo it, you're going to stunt your weight loss progress because your body is going to have to store any calories you consumed as fat while it works on burning all the alcohol away.

So, if you're struggling to lose weight, try cutting out alcohol at least until you have reached your goal weight. At that point, still keep your alcohol intake down to a minimum so that you don't undo all the hard work.

Health Tip #12 – Sleep More

Earlier we talked about how taking days off from your workout to rest is important. It's equally important to make sure you are getting enough quality rest each night. While you are sleeping, your body is hard at work repairing muscles and just generally getting your body back up into optimal condition.

If you don't get enough sleep at night, your metabolism will be slowed down for the entire day. At the same time that your metabolism slows down, your cravings for sugary foods will increase. By combining a slow metabolism with an increased sugar intake, you are just asking for extra belly fat.

So, a full night of sleep every night is essential if you want to make losing weight easier on yourself during the day. Just by getting enough sleep, you can reduce cravings and speed up your metabolism.

The best way to make sure you get enough sleep is to get yourself on a consistent schedule. Go to bed and wake up at the same time, even on weekends. By keeping your sleeping schedule constant, you will give your body the chance to get into a biorhythm. This means you will fall asleep more easily at night and wake up feeling more alert and well rested in the morning.

Another way to help regulate your biorhythm is to keep the same bedtime routine. Get ready for bed in the same order each night. This little bedtime ritual will help send the message to your body that it is time to get ready for sleep.

When you first start doing this, you might find it difficult to fall asleep at your new bedtime or to wake up at your new wake up time. But after the first couple days, it will already start to get easier and after a few weeks, you will hardly even need to look at the clock to know it's time to go to sleep, your body will already start to feel tired when it knows it's time for bed.

Health Tip #13 – Eat Peanut Butter

Peanut butter can be a great weight loss tool. It's delicious, satisfying, and packs a powerful nutritious punch. It's a great way to take care of those nagging cravings without giving into the temptation to scarf down a whole bag of chips or candy.

Peanut butter is high in protein, fiber, and unsaturated fats, the holy trinity of health. You need protein to build the muscles that are going to help you burn more calories. You need the fiber to keep your digestive system running smoothly and maximizing your metabolism. And you need the unsaturated fat to help you absorb and use nutrients as well as put your cravings to rest.

It's also an extremely versatile food. For example, you can add a couple tablespoons to a pan of veggies, shrimp, and noodles for a delicious and easy stir-fry. You could also add some peanut butter to a smoothie with banana, spinach, and yogurt. It tastes delicious in sweet and savory dishes so whatever your craving is at the moment, peanut butter can help you get rid of it without packing on weight.

One word of caution before you run out and buy the biggest tub of peanut butter you can find. Many of the popular brands use hydrogenated fats in their peanut butter recipes. This means Trans fats that, you may remember from the chapter on avocados, are your enemies.

Trans fats do lead to weight gain because your body doesn't actually know how to digest or use them so it just stores them as fat until it can figure out what to do with them. For peanut butter to be a weight loss tool, you need to make sure you are getting the natural stuff with unsaturated fats.

Check the package's label for hydrogenated (or partially hydrogenated) oil or fat. Check the nutrition label to see if it contains Trans fats. If it does, leave it on the shelf. Look for a brand that contains no Trans fats.

Health Tip #14 – Boxing Workouts Are Awesome

Boxing may look like a workout for your arms and upper body but it can actually be a great workout for your abs as well. All the twisting and rotating of your torso is using your abdominal muscles.

Plus, boxing is an awesome cardio workout that lets you take out all your pent-up frustrations and energy on a punching bag while getting the high calorie burn of a good cardio workout. At the same time, your abdominal area is getting a strength workout of a lifetime!

Basically, aerobic boxing is targeting belly fat in 3 key ways. First, it's burning calories with cardio. Secondly, it's building ab muscles with strength training. Finally, it's allowing you to take out your stress and frustration.

Stress is another cause of fat gain. Stress particularly adds fat to your belly. This is because of the hormonal processes that stress triggers in your body. By doing a workout like boxing that offers stress reduction and emotional release, you'll lower your stress. Lowering your stress will lower the hormonal processes that lead to belly fat.

Taken altogether, you'll stop packing on stress weight at the same time that you are maximizing the efficiency with which you burn the fat you already have. And you're doing all of that with the power of your fists!

I hope that you are enjoying this book so far, and if you could spare 30 seconds, I would greatly appreciate you leaving a review on Amazon.com.

Top Tips to Firm Up Your Butt & Thighs

Your butt and thighs are going to be harder to tackle than your belly. This is where your body is storing fat for long-term use. The belly fat is usually the first to get added on and one of the first to get burned off.

This means when you first start working out, the belly area is going to be the first to get toned. It will take you a little longer to start seeing results in the butt and thigh area.

But that doesn't mean it's impossible!

With no excess fat left in the abdomen, your body will have no choice but to start using up the extra fat stored on your lower half.

Use the tips in this second part of the book in order to make sure you are doing everything you can to speed up the process of losing weight and toning your butt and thigh area.

Health Tip #15 – Take the Stairs

Stairs are a godsend for your butt and thighs. It is strength and cardio packed into one *and* it targets your thighs and butt. But you don't need to buy a stair-climbing machine to reap the benefits.

If you take an elevator to get to your office in the morning, take the stairs instead. If you live on one of the upper floors of an apartment complex, start taking the stairs instead of the elevator. Basically, wherever you encounter an elevator, choose to take the stairs instead.

This will provide you a good, quick workout without needing to rearrange your entire schedule. If you don't usually have access to a flight of stairs in your normal life, you should consider getting a stair-climbing machine.

You can keep one in your living room and use it while you watch TV, read a book, or work on finishing up a project for work.

Health Tip #16 – Special Trainers

Your shoes can either be helping or hindering your workout. A bad pair of tennis shoes will only make matters worse. You need a good, quality pair to make sure that your feet are getting the support they need so that you can walk, run, or hike properly.

With a bad pair of tennis shoes, your legs aren't going to be using the right muscles for walking. They'll be focused on compensating for the lack of support.

You can go one step further by getting a pair that is specifically designed to help tone your butt and thighs. Many shoe stores will sell these.

For your butt and thighs, you want a shoe with a specialized sole. The toe will be raised higher up than the heel so that the muscles running up your thighs and butt need to work a little harder with each step.

This won't make walking impossibly difficult. It will just give your butt and thighs a little extra workout with each step so that even when you are taking a rest day or don't have time for a workout, you are still working to tone your backside.

Health Tip #17 – You Must Weight Train

Weight training or strength training is essential for weight loss—especially for the trickier fat around the butt and thighs. Many women shy away from weight training because they assume they'll turn into those big bulky body builders.

But this is not the case. Getting that bulky actually takes a lot of work and conscious effort to pack on mass. Regular weight training will not turn you into a gigantic body builder. What it will do is tone, shape, and firm all that flab and sag you are dealing with.

Weight or strength training works by accomplishing three things.

First, it burns calories. It doesn't burn as many calories as cardio does but its long-term calorie-burning effects are amazing. Weight training kick starts your metabolism. After a workout, your metabolism will stay elevated for 16 hours.

So, if you do your weight training in the morning, you'll burn more calories during the rest of the day.

Secondly, weight-training builds up muscle mass. No, it doesn't bulk you up. It will only do that if you adopt a very rigorous diet and exercise regimen that is designed for bulking up. But it will add just enough muscle to give you that shapely, firm figure you have been dreaming of.

Finally, that added muscle mass will help you lose even more weight!

This is because muscles are more "expensive" than fat. That is to say, they require more calories just to maintain them than fat does.

Fat can be stored without much effort but your body constantly uses up energy to deliver nutrients to your muscles and to make constant minor repairs and modifications.

So, you don't have to focus exclusively on weight training, but do make sure it is a part of your workout plan. You can alternative between weight training and cardio, for example.

You can also combine both into a single workout session by spending the first half doing cardio and the second half doing weight training.

Health Tip #18 – Squats, The Best Workout

Squats are definitely your best choice when it comes to toning and shaping your butt and thighs. This move really targets all the muscles groups involved.

The other advantage is that you don't need any equipment at all to do them. You just need your own two legs. So, you can do them anywhere at any time. If you've got a 10-minute break, shut your office door and do some squats.

The very first tip in this book about focusing on variety rather than number of reps definitely applies here as well. It's better to do a few different workouts in one session than just focusing on doing as many squat reps as you can.

So definitely make sure you use squats but don't neglect the other workouts that are helpful as well. In part three of this book, you'll get 10 workouts that melt away the fat around your butt and thighs and help to tone and shape the muscles in that area as well.

Health Tip #19 – Lunges, the 2nd Best Workout

After squats, lunges are the next best workout for your troublesome butt and thigh area. Lunges help to shape the full area by working the top and bottom of the thigh at the same time.

It also helps shape your butt by developing the muscles that stretch from the top of your butt down to the back of your knee.

Lunges work this entire area beautifully and simply and, just as with squats, you don't need any equipment at all. All the power of this workout comes from your own body.

So, for the best results, combine lunges and squats with one or two other workouts to create a well-rounded and complete workout for your butt and thigh area.

If you're trying to lose fat in your belly, butt, *and* thighs, you should pick workouts that target all the key areas. Squats and lunges will cover your lower half. You can incorporate sit-ups or crunches to tone your upper half.

Use the suggestions in part three to help you craft the perfect workout for your needs.

Health Tip #20 – Step-Ups, The 3rd Best Workout

Step-ups are a way to get the benefits of stair climbing when you don't have access to any stairs (or a stair climbing machine).

Step-ups are more effective than just walking or running when it comes to your butt and thigh area.

This is because the upward movement means that the power has to come from your upper legs (thighs and butt) rather than your calves.

It also adds a strength-training element because you are not just pushing yourself forward but pulling your body weight up with each step.

If you are doing a workout that exclusively targets your butt and thighs, step-ups should definitely be a part of it, especially if you don't have a stair-climbing machine or a staircase.

Health Tip #21 – Join A Class

Gyms and community centers often offer many great classes that can help you burn fat and tone your figure. In most cases, they even offer specialized classes that target the exact areas you are trying to target (like the butt and thighs).

Classes are a great option if you are having trouble staying motivated. If you join a class, you will be less likely to skip a workout or make excuses.

Your teacher and the other class participants can help keep you motivated to accomplish your weight loss goals. You can also talk with them to learn additional tricks for weight loss.

It doesn't hurt that you'll have to pay for the class. You're not going to ditch if you know it's your own money you're wasting!

So, check out what classes are available in your area and try something out. You can even take a risk on an activity you might never have considered before. Trying new things is the best way to find new favorites!

Health Tip #22 – Cardio with A Twist

Cardio is appreciated for its fat burning power. While it's going to burn the fat in your stomach first (as we talked about earlier in this book), it's still great to get in the habit of doing cardio to burn all your fat.

You can also modify your cardio to be more specifically geared toward toning and shaping the butt and thigh area. Earlier, when you read about doing step ups, you learned about the benefits of doing a workout that causes you to pull your body weight upward (instead of just pushing it straight forward).

If you're on a treadmill or elliptical, adjust the incline so that you are running uphill. If you are outdoors, look for a hill or road with a gradual incline and run up that.

The incline will work for the same reason that stair climbing or step-ups work. You are pulling your body weight upward at the same time that you are doing cardio. The muscles that are used to pull your body up an incline are located in your butt and thigh area.

So, increasing the incline on your treadmill or elliptical is the best way to make sure that you are targeting your problem areas with your cardio workout.

Health Tip #23 – Try New Workouts

It's important to try new workouts often. First of all, if you do the same thing day in and day out, you'll hit a weight loss/muscle building plateau where you just start maintaining your current weight and muscle tone because your body has adapted to the workout.

If you have already reached your goal figure at this point, then maybe that's what you're looking for but otherwise, you're going to want to change things up.

The other advantage to new workouts is that they keep your exercise plan interesting. Doing the same thing gets boring but if you change things up once in a while, your workout will continue to be an adventure.

Trying new things is also the best way to figure out what your favorite workouts are. Try something you would have never thought to try before. It might end up being your new favorite hobby!

Health Tip #24 – The BEST Workouts For YOU

Broken up into a few sections, here are the best workouts to melt belly fat and shape your abs. You'll also get the best workouts for toning and firming your butt & thighs.

Don't just pick one workout from each.

Try them all and do them in different combinations so that you can keep your workout fresh and interesting while making sure that you are targeting all the key muscle groups instead of just focusing on one part.

Top 10 Belly Workouts

1. **Sit Ups**

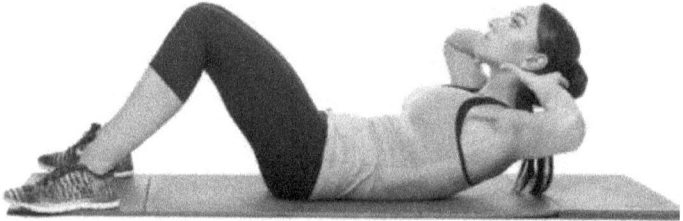

Sit-ups are very simple. Start by lying down on your back with your knees bent and your feet flat on the floor.

Clasp your hands behind your head. Lift yourself up by pivoting from the waist not the neck! Come all the way up to your thighs and then go back down.

Repeat for as many repetitions as you can.

2. Twist Crunches

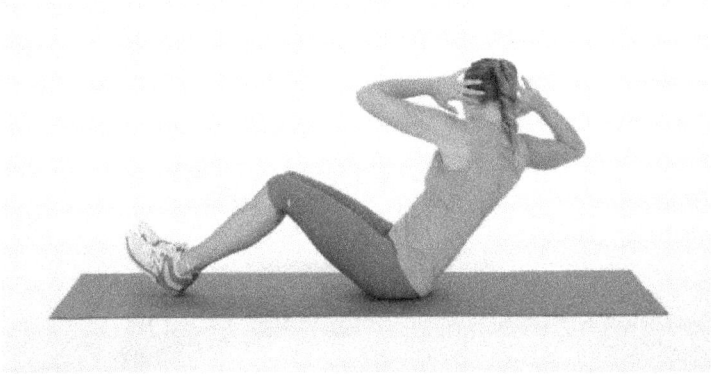

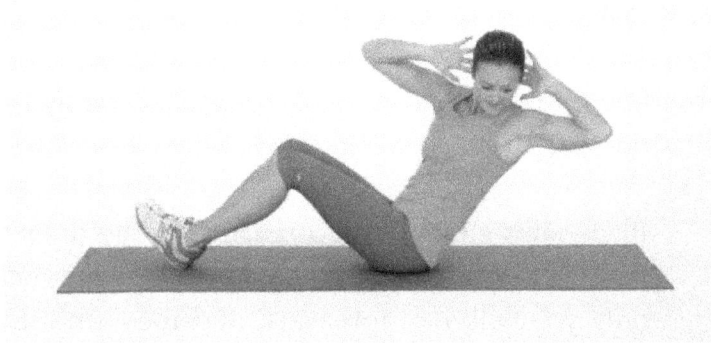

These are like regular crunches except that when you come up, you turn toward one side.

The first time you come up, twist and aim toward your left leg. Then go back down. When you come up again, twist and aim toward your right leg.

Repeat this for as many repetitions as you can.

3. Plank Twists

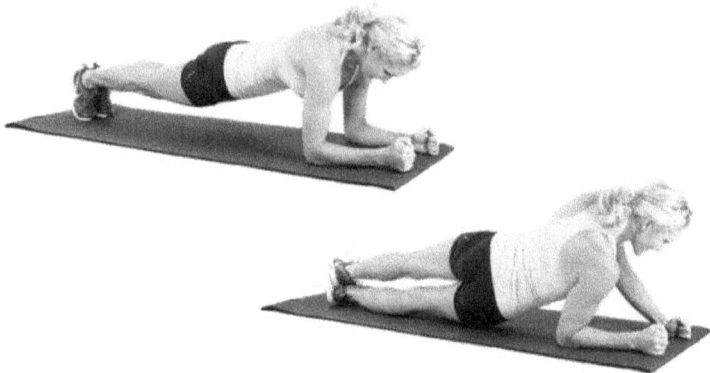

Get into plank position. To do this, start by lying down on your stomach.

Place your elbows and forearms on the floor and clasp your hands together. Push up onto your toes so that only your elbows, forearms, and toes are touching the floor. Keep your body straight (like a plank).

While in this position, twist your core to the left. Keep your shoulders straight and your toes firmly pressed into the floor so that only your stomach and thighs are facing to the left.

You want all the movement and power to be coming from your core. Twist your torso all the way to your right. Repeat for as many repetitions as you can.

4. Leg Lifts

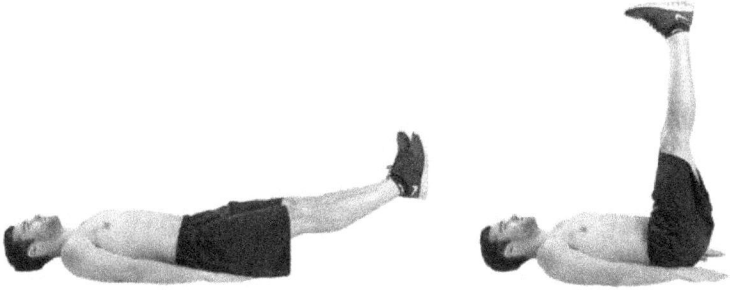

Lie down on your back with your legs straight and your toes pointed.

Keep your upper body flat against the floor as you lift your legs up off the ground.

Lift with your core. Do not bend your knees.

5. V Lifts

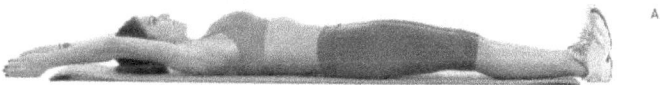

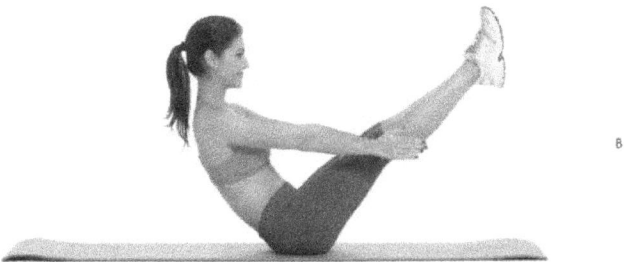

This is similar to the leg lifts except that as you are lifting up your legs, you will also lift up your torso.

Don't bend your knees or your spine. As you lift up, you will form a straight V shape.

You can either have your arms straight up above your head or lift them out in front of you (so that you'll look more like an upside-down A than a V).

6. Donkey Kicks

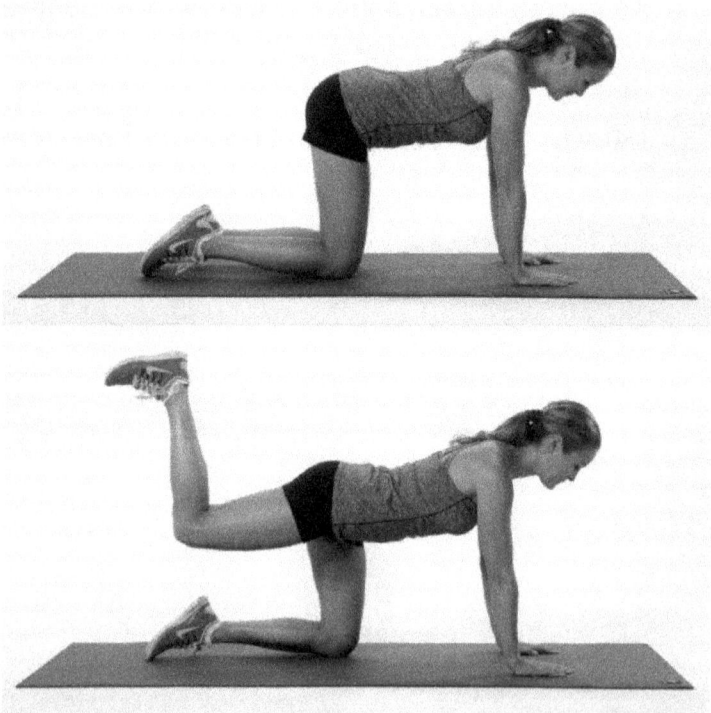

Start in a push up position with your arms straight. Don't lock your elbows.

Lift your right leg off the floor and then bend your knee up and in toward your chest. Then, kick it back out.

Without lowering it back down to the floor, repeat this for as many repetitions. Then, switch legs and do it with the other leg.

7. Boat Pose

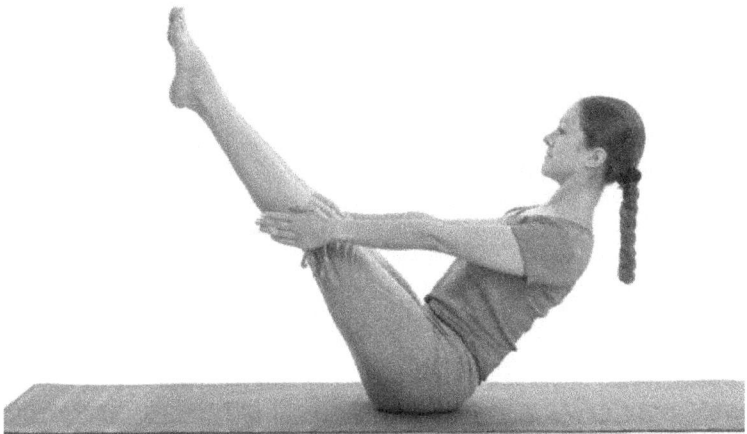

This is just like the V Lift workout described above except that instead of doing repetitions, you maintain the V shape pose consistently.

Holding the pose builds strength and endurance in your abdominal muscles.

8. Plank Pose

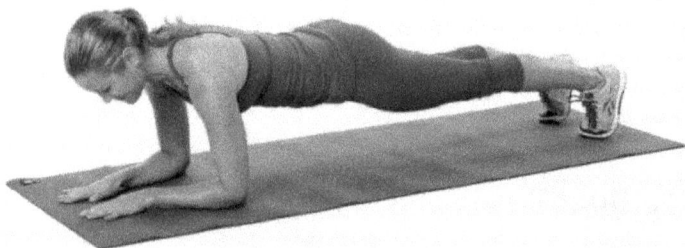

This is like the plank position described above in "plank twists" except that instead of twisting, you simply hold the plank pose.

Focus on tightening your core and make sure that you keep your body in a flat plank position. Your butt may start to rise up in the air.

Make sure to pull it back down.

9. Leg Swings

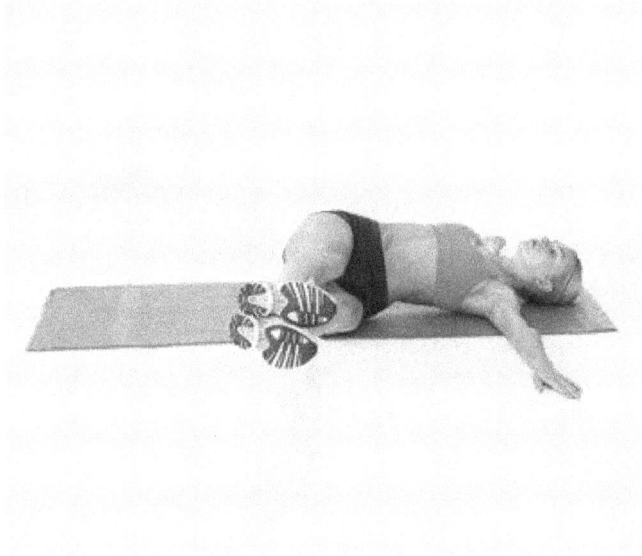

Lie down on your back with your legs straight. Raise your legs up so that your toes are pointing toward the ceiling and your legs form a 90° angle with your torso.

Lower your legs to the left side (while maintaining the 90° angle). You might not be able to reach the floor. That's ok. Raise them back up and then lower to them the right side. Imagine your legs are the swinging pendulum of a clock.

Use your core to pivot your hips and move your legs from side to side.

10. Forward Bends

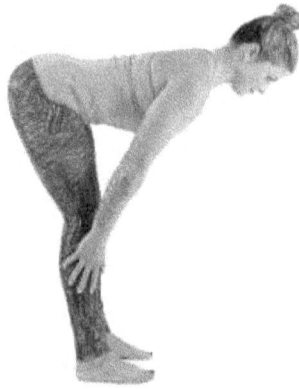

This is like doing sit ups while standing.

Start by standing up straight with your feet placed hip width apart. Cross your arms over your chest.

Slowly bend your torso down toward the floor. Keep your spine straight and make sure that you are bending at the waist (not just dropping your shoulders).

Once your torso is parallel with the floor, pull yourself back up. Again, pivot from the waist, not your shoulders or neck. Repeat as many times as you can.

Top 10 Butt & Thigh Workouts

1. Squats

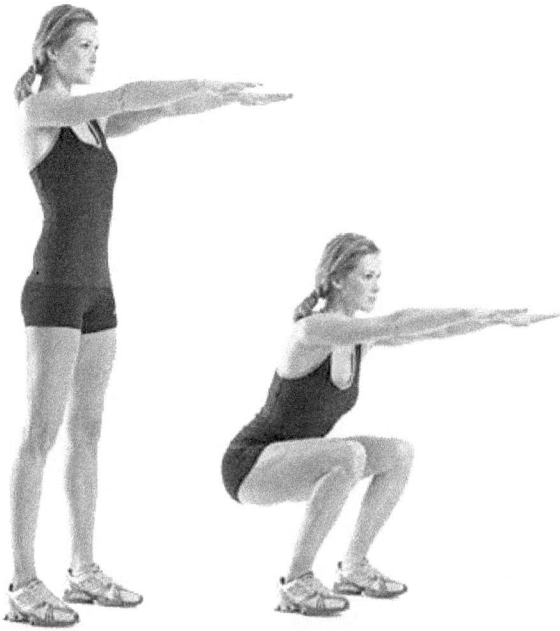

To do a squat, stand with your feet wider than hip width apart.

While keeping your upper body straight, bend until your knees form a 90° angle. Hold this pose as long as you can.

2. Lunges

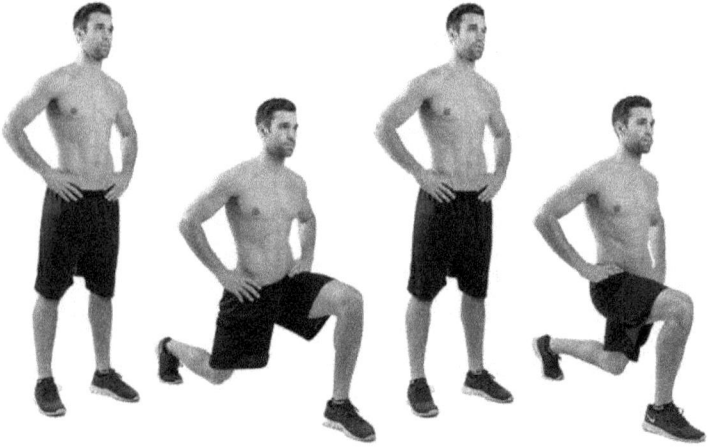

Start by standing with your feet hip width apart. Step out with your left leg and bend your left knee until you are in lunge position.

Hold and then stand back up to repeat with the right leg.

3. **Step Ups**

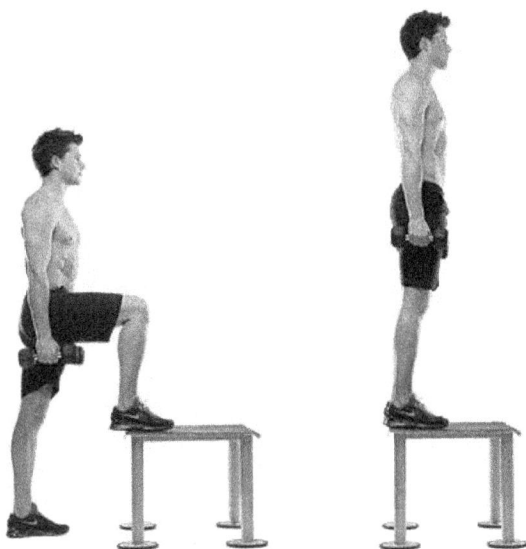

Use a sturdy box or chair or the bottom step of a staircase. Stand in front of it.

Without bending your spine or using your torso at all, step up with the left leg. Then bring the right leg up. Step your left leg back down on the floor behind you and then bring your right leg down.

Repeat with your right leg.

4. Stair Climbing

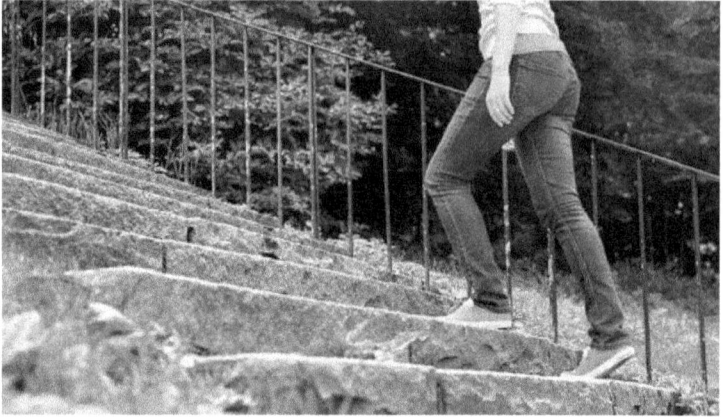

Climb up stairs or use a stair-climbing machine. Go up and down multiple times. You can skip two or three steps at a time if you are capable.

5. Incline Running

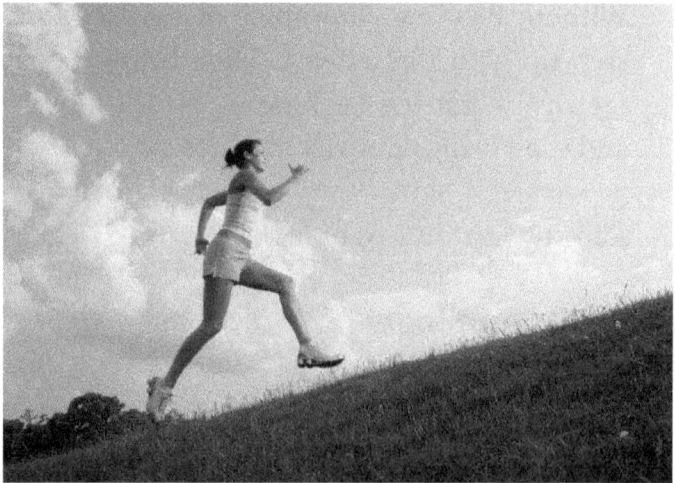

Increase the incline on your treadmill or elliptical (or find a road outside with an incline) and run at your full power.

As you read earlier, the incline will tone your butt and thighs.

6. Chair Pose

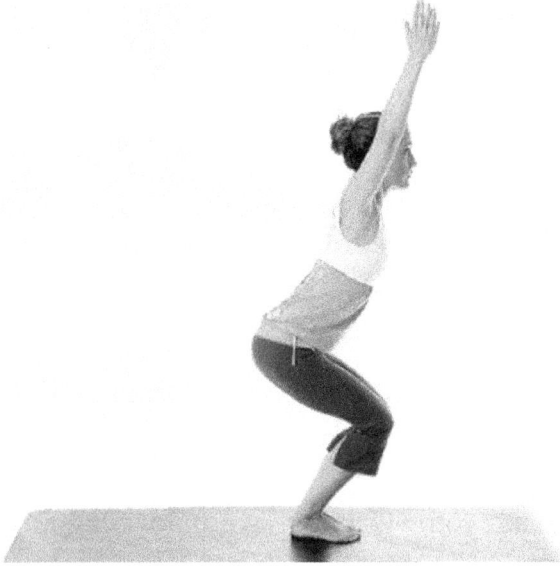

Start with your feet hip width apart. Raise your arms above your head and bend your torso forward very slightly. Keep your spine straight.

Drop your hips down and bend at the knees (as if you were going to sit in a chair). Hold this as long as you can.

7. Brave Warrior Pose

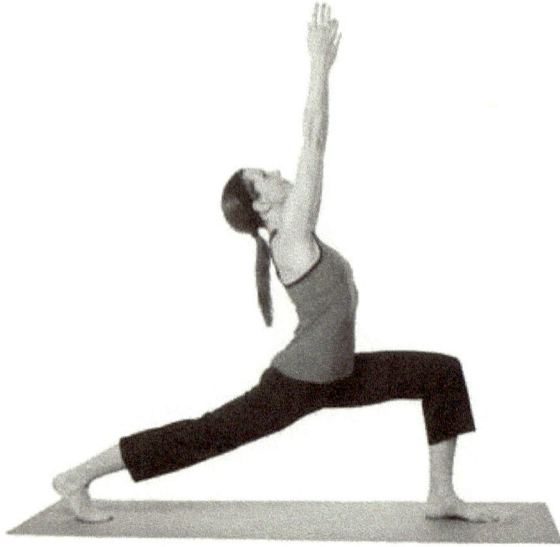

This one is challenging for beginners. Stand with your feet hip width apart.

Raise your arms above your head. Carefully bend forward at the waist. Keep your spine straight.

As you bend your torso forward to be parallel with the ground, raise your left leg behind you and point your toes straight back behind you.

You'll form a sort of T shape while balancing on one leg. Hold this as long as you can and then repeat on the other leg.

8. Standing Leg Lifts

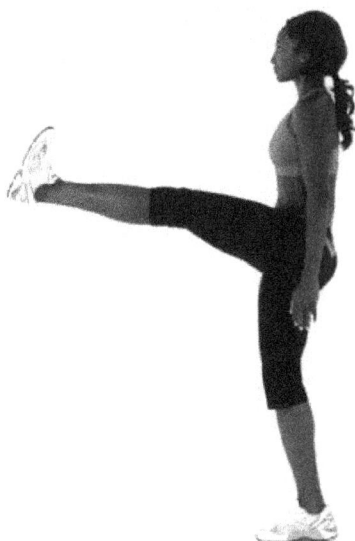

Stand straight with your feet hip width apart. Keep your knees straight but not locked.

Raise your left leg out in front of you as far up as you can without bending your knee.

Bring it back down. Repeat the move with the other leg.

9. Reverse Leg Lifts

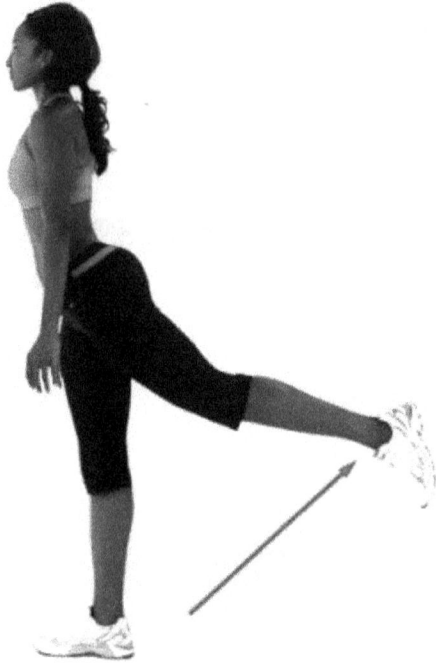

This is similar to the leg lifts above except that instead of raising your leg in front of you, you raise it out behind you.

Go as far back as you can without bending your knee.

Alternate between lifting your left and right leg.

10. Jumping Squats

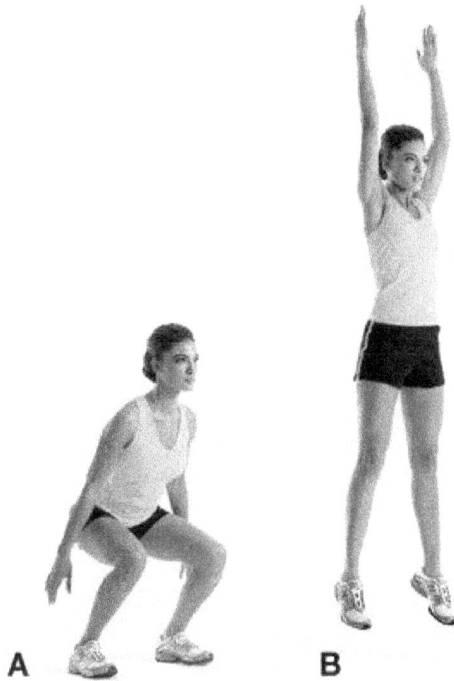

A   B

Get into the squat position described in the first workout.

Then, jump up into the air while raising your arms above your head.

Make sure that the power for the jump is coming from your thighs, not your upper body.

When you land back on the ground, immediately go back into squat position. Do as many repetitions as you can.

Once again, thank you for reading this book, and I hope you're getting a lot of valuable information. I would greatly appreciate it if you could take 30 seconds to leave me a review for this book on Amazon.com.

Top Tips to BOOST Overall Health

For women, multitasking is a norm. For women who work, especially, it is really hard to find any time to take care of their health and maintain a body that is fit.

It does not always have to be several hours at the gym or at a class to get in shape. There are simple things that you can do yourself, in the comfort of your home to achieve the body that you always dream of.

There are only two things that you absolutely need; the right method, and the motivation. With this in place, there is no reason why you cannot fit a healthy routine into your extremely busy one. All you need to know are some simple tricks to make this transformation easier.

This book is ideal for anyone who is struggling to get started and stick on to one fitness plan that works. You will learn all about eating right and simple modules that you can choose in order to get the results that you want.

I have very carefully chosen tips and tricks that will work for women who are working or have a busy day just managing their homes. Now all you need to do is kick off the good habits and make sure that you stay motivated enough to stick to them.

If you can just follow these tips diligently, I can assure you that you that the results that you get will be motivation enough to keep going.

I wish you all a great start and a healthy life ahead. I hope that this book is of good use to you. All you need to do is incorporate these tips gradually in your life and you will most certainly see a big difference physically and also mentally.

Health Tip #25 – Increase Physical Activity

The biggest problem that most of us face is that a large part of the day is spent in a sedentary manner. We also have so many devices that very tactfully reduce the amount of effort that we put into things.

As a result, we become more lethargic and a lot more rigid in our body movements.

The best thing to do when you are starting your fitness routine is to add movement to your regular activities.

So, if you are talking the elevator, swap that with stairs unless you have high blood pressure or trouble with your knees.

Change the channel of the TV without a remote.

Do the dishes yourself or just mop the house.

These activities make up for a type of physical activity called Spontaneous Physical Activity and can help you lose close to 350 more calories every day.

In fitness, every small thing that you do counts. It is all these small routine activities that come together to make you more energetic. You will see that you have the stamina to stay active all day long without any sugar or coffee to keep you going!

Health Tip #26 – Find A Partner

Motivation is something that we all lack. A gym owner that I know said that he dreads the day every member at his gym actually shows up to work out; his facilities would be insufficient then.

This only means that there are many people who get started but lost track somewhere along the way.

The best way to stay motivated is to find a partner who has the same fitness goals as you. You will have the interest to continue for longer when you start with a partner. It is only until you see the results that you need a partner. After that, your results will be your motivation.

You could take your spouse along with you, find a friend who will join you or better still, get a colleague from work to join you.

When you have this sort of support, you see that untimely snacks, take away foods or even that small piece of chocolate is easier to resist.

You will also be able to 'share the guilt' on days that you choose to binge. The idea is to monitor one another and ensure that you are both on the road to a healthier life. You can do all of this alone, but a partner just makes it easier.

Health Tip #27 – Eat with Your Mind

Research shows that our inability to stick to a good diet is all in the mind. Of course, we have all heard about the lack of will power to continue with a good diet. However, what is more important is our perception of food.

Many people fail in following good eating habits because they believe that certain foods are "not enough" for them. For instance, when you are eating a nice lettuce salad, you think that the meal is light and hence the body reacts the same way.

When you think that a certain portion or type of food is not enough, the body produces a hormone called ghrelin that does not let you feel full.

What really works is putting your mind into the foods that are more calorific. This includes nuts, avocado or even proteins like fish or shrimp.

When you approach food in this manner, you are able to choose healthier options like a good and nutritious broth, a vegetable and shrimp salad etc. You will notice how these foods begin to feel like a real treat. So, when you are starting out with any diet plan, do it with optimism and an open mind.

Health Tip #28 – Turn Off The TV

Studies have revealed alarming correlations between the time a person spends watching TV and his weight. People who are obese are known to watch a lot of TV.

So, for starters, it would be a great idea to stop eating while you watch television.

According to recent reports, your chances of being obese increase by 23% for every 2 hours that you spend before the television.

In addition to that, you also consume more calories unknowingly. This is not a small amount of calories but a whopping 280 of them! So, the next time you head to the living room with a plate of food, think again.

You see, TV also eats into the time that you could have spent sleeping or perhaps, working out.

It may not be easy to say goodbye to the TV altogether but it is a good idea to start slowly. For instance, you can try to incorporate the "ten-minute work out" that we will discuss in the following chapter between your favorite TV show.

Slowly work your way up to swapping an hour of TV with exercise. Also, try to have all your meals at the table to avoid over eating and to also be able to eat mindfully.

Health Tip #29 – Eat All Your Meals

This is extremely important for busy women who tend to skip their breakfast because they do not have the time. Well you could even eat a few fruits and some bread for breakfast but never skip a meal.

When you get into the habit of skipping meals, there are two results that you can expect. Firstly, your cravings for foods that are high in sugar and fat will increase.

This is because your body needs instant energy to make up for the meal that you skipped. So, this will naturally make you want to binge and eat everything you are not supposed to.

Second, your body goes into a conservation mode. When you constantly deprive your body of the right amount of food, you brain perceives this as an emergency.

The brain tells the rest of your body that the availability of food is limited. So, there is a need to fight and survive. As a result, the fat storage in the body increases.

Your body is only doing this to safeguard you from starvation. However, the resulting effect is totally contrary to what you want to achieve. So, it is always important to eat well, especially when you are training.

Health Tip #30 – Get Yourself a New Plate

As surprising or uncanny as this may seem, you can actually control the amount of food that you consume by changing the color of the plate that you are currently eating from.

If the color of the plate and your food are contrasting, you tend to eat lesser.

This has been proved by a study at Cornell University, which showed that your serving size reduces by 20% when the color of the plate is a contrast to the food that you are eating.

So, if you are having trouble controlling the dessert intake, you can just eat out of a blue plate. This combination is a natural suppressant for your appetite. As weird as this may sound to you, it has been proved scientifically and that makes it reason enough to give it a shot.

Health Tip #31 – Find A Goal

When you start, you need to have a goal. Without that, your exercise regime and your eating habits will lack direction.

The way you work out or eat when you want to drop the extra pounds is drastically different from the way you would eat when you want to just tone up all the muscles in the body. This principal applies to your exercise regime as well.

So, when you begin, identify your goals. If needed, you can also note them down like a checklist that you actually tick off as you achieve the goals. Make short-term goals and break down your long-term goals as well. This makes your goals easier to achieve.

With every goal that you tick off on your check list, you will see that you have more energy and more willingness to face any challenge that is put before you. You will only get better each day.

So instead of saying "I will lose 100 pounds", tell yourself, "I will do one more rep tomorrow". Weight loss is the side effect of a good workout and diet plan.

Enjoying this book?

Check out my other best sellers!

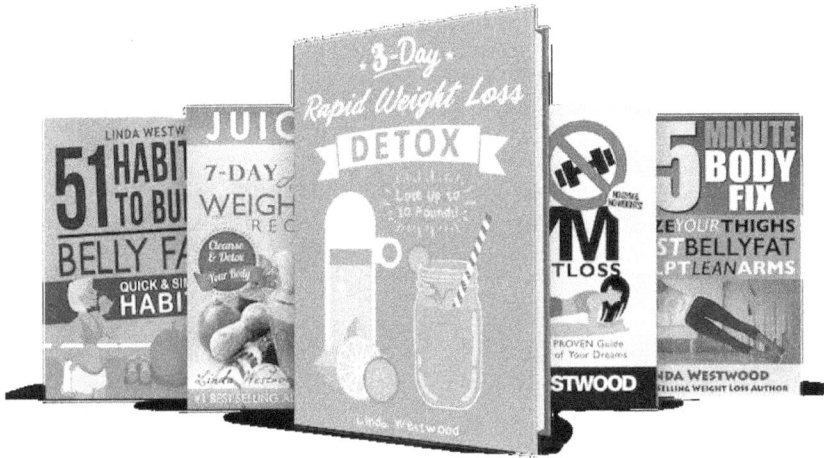

Get your next book on sale here:

TopFitnessAdvice.com/go/books

Top Fitness Tips to Get You RESULTS Fast

In order to get completely fit, there are no short cuts. Yes, there are shorter, more time-based regimes but nothing that you can count as a quick fix.

You need to exercise for your body to become efficient. When the body becomes efficient, it works in your favor. Your metabolism increases.

You are able to absorb nutrition better and burn the excess fat better, too. So, there is no turning away from exercise if you truly desire a body that is toned and fit.

Health Tip #32 – Find A Routine That Suits You

The worst thing you can do with exercising is get stuck in a workout that is boring. That will kill half the motivation and you will have to work really hard to get yourself to continue it.

So, what you need to do is find a routine that will suit your interest. This could be a Zumba session after work, a nice dip in the pool in the morning or even a good run.

If you are someone who loves to train at the gym, there is no reason why you should not do it.

If you are on a weight loss program, it is a good idea to choose workouts that are of moderate or high intensity depending upon your abilities.

Health Tip #33 – Interval Training Is a Good Idea

If you simply love your cardio training, you may want to try interval training.

When you practice this type of training, you will lose only fat and not too much muscle (this definitely minimizes it). If you start losing muscle, you will notice that you feel tired really easily and you look unhealthily skinny. Instead work towards optimizing fat loss with this kind of training program.

For instance, if you choose sprinting as your work out module, then it is a good idea to go all out for about a minute and then slow it down for about two minutes.

This gives you a fat blast regime and it is recommended that you follow this for about three days each week.

Another excellent way to practice interval workout is to choose pilates. In one hour of your pilates workout, you can include several variations to make your routine more effective. This means you have the option of speeding up or slowing down a particular exercise.

You can also alter the resistance that you have in each exercise. This sort of high intensity interval routine is most recommended for busy individuals who do not have more than 30 minutes to spare in a day for their exercise routine.

Health Tip #34 – Don't Be Afraid to Lift Weights

Ladies, if you think that you will look muscular and manly by pushing weights, then here is something that you need to know.

It takes a lot of effort and very precise training to build the kind of muscle that you see on body builders. If you add resistance to your exercises in the form of weights, you will notice that the effects are better and faster.

There is a scientific and quite a logical reason for this. People who have larger muscle mass tend to burn more calories. So, if you can combine strength training with cardio training, the results are faster and long lasting. You do not have to work on a very long routine. About 20 minutes of strength training is good enough.

Since your goat is not to bulk up, you need not push extremely heavy weights. What you need to work on is improving the quality o your muscles while increasing the muscle mass in the process.

If you do not want to invest in a gym or in weights, you can even use a resistance band to increase your strength and overall muscle mass with a simple routine.

Health Tip #35 – Stretching Is Important

When you follow any kind of workout routine, there is going to be a certain amount of strain on your muscle. This produces lactic acid that is responsible for the soreness that you feel after a hard workout routine.

If you want your muscles to be relaxed, you have to remember to stretch. If you choose to dedicate two days to stretching with a routine like yoga, it will do you good.

But remember to stretch EVERY DAY after you are done with your workout.

This is the only way to ensure that you have the strength to continue training. If you feel extremely sore, there is no way you will be able to work to your best capacity the following day.

Stretch the muscles that you have used. For instance, if you have done a ten-minute routine that includes mountain runners, planks and push-ups, you need to stretch the shoulders and your abdomen muscles as they have been worked the most.

So, understand what muscle or what part of the body you are working out for the best possible results.

Health Tip #36 – Let Your Muscles Work

No matter what workout plan you choose for toning, make sure that you put different muscles on the job. When a larger group of muscles are at work, you are definitely going to burn more calories.

So, squats followed by shoulder press, burpees, etc., are the perfect work out options for ladies.

Health Tip #37 – Make the Most Out of Technology

You don't have to be with a personal trainer to keep a track of what workout you are doing. In fact, with superior technology, you can manage even without a trainer.

There are several apps that can do multiple things for you each time.

From scheduling your workout to giving you tips to keep your posture correct you have applications that can do everything for you. So, no matter where you are travelling to, you can always take your trainer along.

Some applications also allow you to join a fitness forum or group where your results can be shared with others and vice versa. This is a great way to keep yourself motivated to continue with your regime.

You will also find several accessories like stop clocks, workout charts etc. that make it easier to manage any routine that you are following. Even if your routine is just a simple jog in the park, there are apps that can calculate your progress rather effectively.

Health Tip #38 – Keep Calm

This is the most important fitness and toning regime for you. For busy women, especially, there are so many things to take care of that it may take its toll on you.

Sometimes, you may even end up feeling over worked and stressed. That is when you must put in additional efforts to keep yourself calm and composed.

Try activities like meditation to help you. You can even choose to use alternate therapies like aromatherapy, massages or even movement therapy to get rid of all the stress that you are putting on yourself.

Now, you are probably wondering what the relationship between weight and stress is. Well, when the stress level in the body increases, a certain type of hormone called cortisone is released. This hormone is responsible for the storage of fat in our body.

So, relaxing, getting good sleep and steering clear of stress will actually work to your advantage in more ways than one. And, if all fails just remember to breathe focus on the things that actually matter to you.

Health Tip #39 – If You Skip, Make Up

It is inevitable to miss a day of exercising. You were probably too tired from work or you probably had an important meeting to attend. In such cases, don't beat yourself up. Instead, try to make up for this missed session.

If you know that you are going to miss you exercise someday, you can make up by making yourself more physically active that day. This means squats as you clean your teeth, calf muscle exercises if you are waiting in a queue or using the bathroom on a higher floor in order to ensure you have to take the stairs.

You can also make up for missing exercise by ensuring that you continue the very next day. The problem with missing a day of exercise is that it becomes very hard to get back to the rhythm unless you have been at it for a really long time.

When you are out on a holiday, try to set 10 or 15 minutes aside to do something simple like running or skipping. That way, you are able to stay focused and you will not find yourself too lazy to get back to the routine that you have set for yourself after you get home from a vacation.

Health Tip #40 – Challenge Yourself

As you get stronger, you will body will demand more. So, whatever your fitness plan is, make sure you keep challenging yourself.

If you are comfortable doing three laps when you are swimming, try pushing it to one more lap. If you love your cardio routine, add five minutes to your current time.

These small increments will give you results faster than you expect. Of course, it does not mean that you keep on increasing your laps till you go to 100. You can challenge yourself in more ways than you think.

Simple things like adding more resistance, changing the pattern of working out and even reducing resting time between sets can make your body stronger, more active and give you high endurance.

Remember never to get stagnant. It is not only boring but is also the easiest way to slow your progress down. If you follow a fitness idol, you will see that he or she keeps experimenting with different combinations and modules. This makes each day more fun as you have something new to look forward to.

In this process, you may even find something new that is easier and more interesting for you. So, remember, the best way to stay in that progressive stage of weight loss is to keep yourself on your toes.

Health Tip #41 – Try Bodyweight Training

There is no weight under the sun that can give you better results than the weight of your own body.

Calisthenics is a very popular form of exercise that is getting noticed these days by everyone. These exercises not only tone you up faster but also make you a lot stronger that you will ever be by lifting the heaviest weights.

Even some intense forms of yoga like Ashtanga yoga give you the benefit of using your own body weight to get better results. With this type of training you will notice that the additional health benefits are also many.

Exercises like planks, mountain climbers, burpees and many more engage your entire body while giving you the results that you want.

But you need to make sure that your postures are correct and that you take it one step at a time with these exercises. They are harder to execute and hence require a lot more care.

Health Tip #42 – Stay Committed to Goals

Do not waver from "I want to have fab abs" to "I want great legs" each day. Choose a fitness routine that will give you over all benefits and be clear of your goals. Weight loss is the added perk that you get for exercising. So, you don't have to always worry about that.

The best thing to do would be to choose goals that can be of maximum benefit to you overall. When you set your fitness goals, try to do it with an expert. That is when you will have more success.

For example, most women want to reduce belly fat like it is some epidemic.

But, if you have a weak lower back and you are doing 100 crunches each day, you are more likely to have injuries and pain. In these cases, your goal should be to strengthen the weak body part before you move on to losing weight.

So, a good thing to do would be to consult an expert, get the right understanding of your body and then proceed to make goals.

That is when you will be able to commit to these goals better. The reason is that wrong goals can hinder results and demotivate you.

Set long term and short-term goals and stick to them. Like I said before, achieving your short-term goals will motivate you and help you stick to your goals much better.

Health Tip #43 – Try 10-Minute Routines

There are several ten-minute routines that are available on the Internet. You may try one of them based on your requirements. These routines are high intensity short duration activities that will help you burn fat and tone your body at the same time.

When you are practicing a routine from a CD or the Internet, be mindful of the posture. The slightest mistake may cause injuries and you will have no one to hold responsible for it but yourself.

If you have friends who work out regularly or even professionally, seek advice at all times to keep yourself safe.

Here is a ten-minute routine that you can try and the only equipment you need is a resistance band.

- 2 sets of push-ups with your knees bent

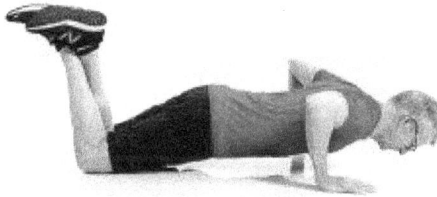

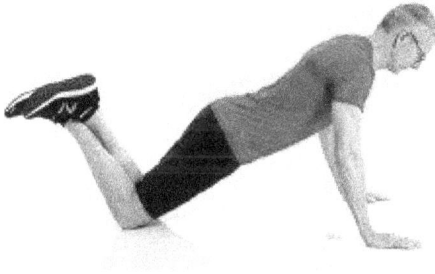

- 2 sets of tricep dips

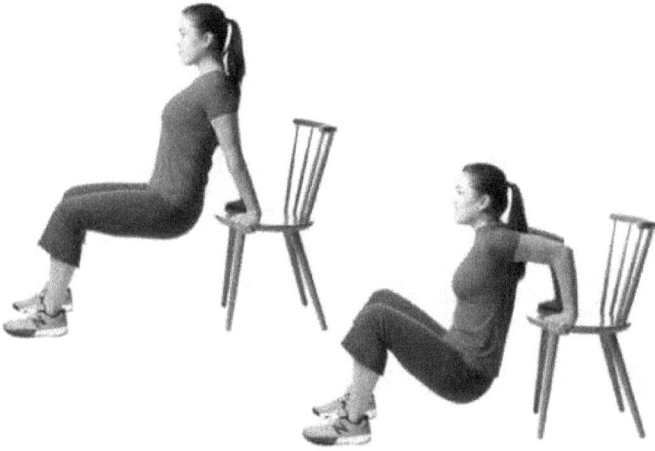

- 1 set on either side of Shoulder press with resistance band

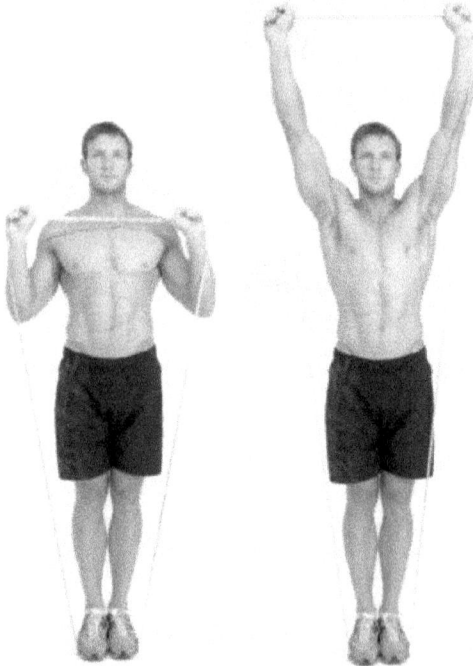

- 2 sets of shoulder press with lunge

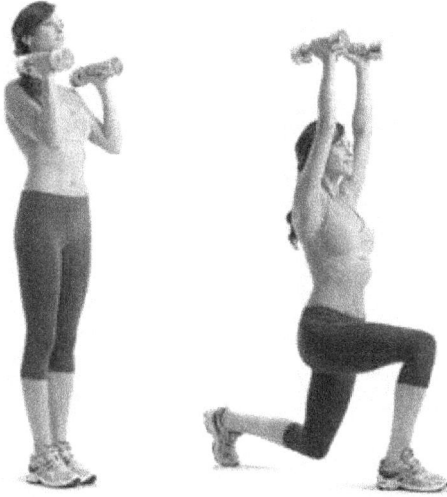

- 2 sets of bicep curls with resistance band

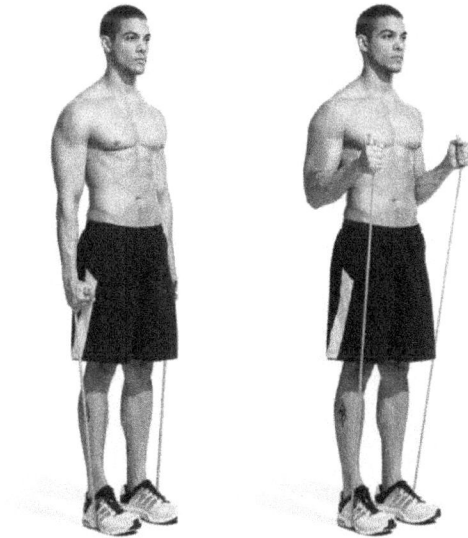

- 2 sets of lateral raises with resistance band

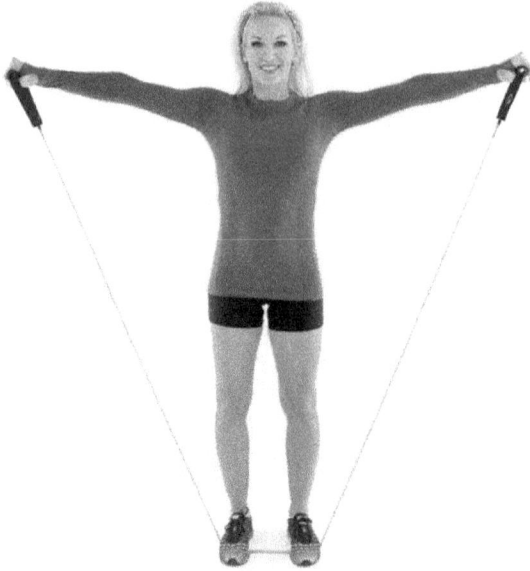

- 2 sets of squats

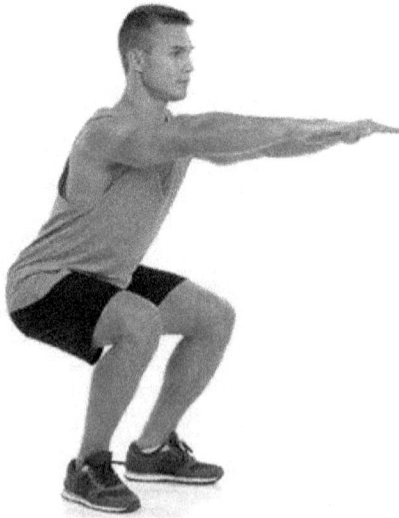

- 1 set of lunges on each side

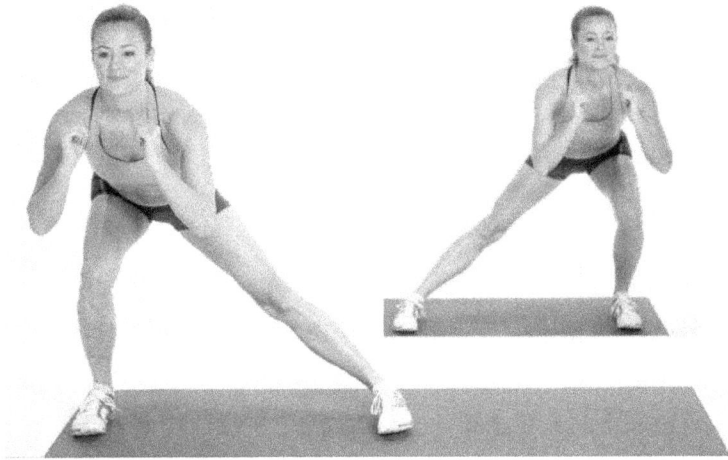

- 2 sets Crunches

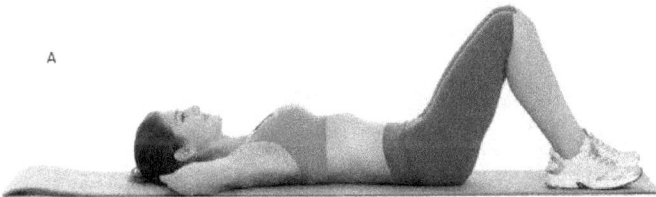

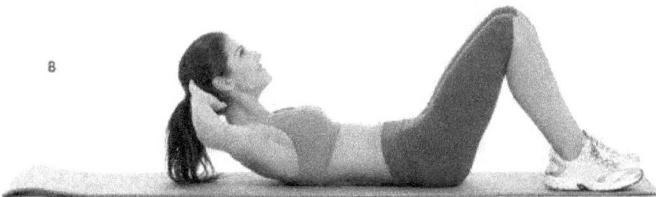

- 2 sets of Back raises

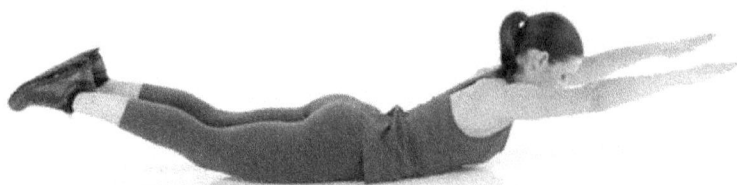

Each set can vary between 12 to 15 repetitions. If you do not know what any exercise means, you will be able to find a detailed description of each of them on the Internet.

Health Tip #44 – Track Your Progress

Unless you know how much better you have become, you will not know how much more you need to do. When you start off, note all your statistics in terms of your weight and inches.

You must weigh yourself every week and measure the inches every month. If you are seeing no difference at all, you may want to consult an expert. Remember that weight is not the only indicator of progress. There are many things that you can measure to see how well your body is doing.

Once you have a great workout routine in place, you have to shift your attention to what you eat. Never go on crash diets or take fat loss pills, as they will work against everything that you are working for.

The next chapter will tell you in complete detail how you can alter your eating habits to suit your goals. The focus is on helping you control those cravings that shake you off your determined weight loss plan. You will notice that it is not so hard to keep your mind off the foods that are not the healthiest choice available.

If you're enjoying this book and would love to let other potential readers know how great it is, please take a few seconds to leave a review on Amazon.com.

Top Tips to Eat Right & Get Healthy FAST

Nutrition forms 70% of your weight loss program. If you think that you can eat all you want because you are working out, then good luck with weight loss.

There is no way your body will work the way you want it to if you constantly fuel it wrongly. This section is dedicated towards helping you eat clean while you train dirty.

It is really not that hard to curb your cravings if you are constantly giving your body the food that it needs.

Health Tip #45 – No Processed Foods, Please!

It is very tempting to give in to processed foods because they are easier to cook and even consume. As busy women, it is common for you to get ready to eat or even microwave foods and get on with it.

These foods can be extremely harmful for your body as they are loaded with several other ingredients that you do not want entering your body. Most of them have even been detected with deadly products like lead in them.

So, for all health reasons, it is a good idea to stay away from these processed foods altogether. It is mostly during snack time that people get carried away by these processed foods.

What you need to know is that these foods are packed with several hydrogenated fats and also contain high levels of sugar. The nutritional value of these products is not even a fraction of your unprocessed foods. So, if you want to eat clean in order to lose weight, you need to make sure that you eat right.

For this, it is a good idea to cook with fresh produce. When you feel hungry, substitute the processed snacks with healthy and energizing options like nuts or celery sticks. That way, you will also ensure better nutrition for your body.

Health Tip #46 – No Crash Diets

This is definitely the worst thing that you can do for yourself. You see, when you suddenly deprive your body of certain foods, it goes into a state of shock.

This means that the brain is telling the rest of your body that you are in a crisis like a drought that is causing the food shortage. Your brain looks at food deprivation as a threat and not as a "weight loss" mechanism.

So, your body is signaled to store as much fat as possible in order to prevent malnutrition or any shock due to lack of a particular nutrient in the body.

As for the fuel that your body needs to function, it begins to eat into your muscle mass. That will leave you feeling tired always. And, the lesser the muscle mass, the fewer calories you can burn.

So, these diets only work opposite to the results that you expect. If you really want to start eating healthy, consult a nutritionist and follow a healthy and natural eating plan for the best results.

Fresh produce, natural foods and lots of liquid are what you really need in order to look and feel healthy. Not eating on time or even skipping meals will only do more damage to your body with time.

Health Tip #47 – Baby Steps First

Following a balanced diet or a healthy diet is a very healthy choice and you must, indeed, be excited to get started. However, it is best that you take these changes one-step at a time.

It takes some time for the body to get used to a certain eating habit and you need to give it that much time.

If you dive head first into a new plan, you will find it very hard to stick to it. Get yourself a diet plan and then divide it into easy and realistic bits that you know you can follow.

You may want to add one healthy bit each day in your diet and replace the existing foods with healthier options. You need to do this one at a time until you know that you will not crave for the bad foods any longer.

If you have sweet cravings at a certain time of the day, choose fruits or raisings as an alternative. If you need to reduce binging or the portion of food that you are consuming, try to drink lots of water. Water will keep you hydrated and will also reduce your appetite in a healthy way.

Health Tip #48 – Know Your Calorie Requirement

On an average a person needs two snacks and three meals on a daily basis. This is the amount that he needs in order to fulfill his caloric value.

But this value changes drastically from one person to the other and you need to know your calorie requirement before you adopt any diet plan.

In most simple terms, you will lose weight when the number of calories that you burn exceeds the number of calories that you consume.

However, you also need a basic amount of calories or energy that your body must have in order to function properly. This is called your daily calorie requirement.

Unless you know this value, you will not be able to calculate how many calories you need to consume and how many you need to burn in order to initiate the weight loss program.

Like most fitness experts say, this is like shooting without a target. Your bullets just go in every direction but do not hit any target.

You will be able to plan your meals much better when you know how much energy you need. That way you will also ensure that you do not deprive your body of what it actually needs.

Health Tip #49 – Volumetrics

This is a very interesting diet practice that saves you a lot of time and gives you the results that you need.

In short, it is the ideal way to measure the food that you consume if you are someone who does not have too much time on her hands.

To help you understand this better, volumetrics is nothing but calculating the calories that you are consuming based on the size of every bite. This helps you eat as much as you want without getting too many calories into your system.

It is just simple math. If the number of calories that you consume per spoon is less, then the portion of the food that you are eating can be bigger.

That way you can eat till you are satiated, which means that you are no longer hungry. But, the best part is that the amount of calories that you consume can still be controlled.

A good way to make sure that you are eating fewer calories in each bite is to eat foods that have a high volume.

This includes fruits, soups and vegetables and reducing the amount of low volume foods that have high levels of calories.

Health Tip #50 – Keep the Diet Flexible

This is especially necessary for women who do not have too much time always. You can make different diet plans that may vary in the contents and the degree of difficulty in preparing.

Of course, variety is extremely necessary if you do not want to be bored to death with your diet plan.

This form of boredom is also responsible for cravings to kick in. So, try to make your diet as much fun as you can.

Also remember that you will make several mistakes in the beginning. It is alright to eat something that you are "not supposed to" when you are still trying to get the hang of the whole concept of dieting.

Don't beat yourself up. Remember, dieting and fitness or even weight loss should be fun.

This also means that you can never be overly disciplined in this process. It is alright to let your hair down and have a good time.

Being happy is a big part of weight loss, remember?

That will curb the cravings, make the overall experience better and also keep you motivated to keep going with your weight loss program.

Health Tip #51 – Kiss the Sugars Goodbye

Sugar, as you must have heard a million times, is the biggest enemy of weight loss. The American Heart Association does not recommend more than 6 teaspoons of additional sugar each day for women. Additional sugar refers to your refined sugars that you add over the sugar that you get from natural foods.

The only problem with sugar is that the sources are undetermined. Almost every condiment that you pick up has some amount of sugar that you are probably unaware of. So, be sure to read the labels of foods that you buy.

You see, because of this hidden sugar the amount that a person consumes on an average is very high. This the primary reason for several weight related issues.

Stay away from artificial sweeteners and refined sugars as much as you can. With candy and cake, you know that it is there but you could be consuming unwanted sugars through other products. So, take as much care as you can.

If you do have sweet cravings, look for healthier alternatives like fruits. Wouldn't you pick juicy strawberries over a bar of candy? I would!

It is not just healthy but lip smackingly tasty as well. There are so many other alternatives like raisins and dates that work just as well.

Health Tip #52 – High Quality Proteins Are a Must

Never compromise on your proteins. They do a lot for your body. If you are a woman who needs all her energy to get through her day, then, you cannot do without proteins.

You see, proteins are responsible for all the repairing processes that occur in our body.

When you work out, your muscles develop small tears and strains. This is true even if you do not lift weights. So, you need to fuel your body with high quality proteins that will take care of any damage.

There is more to protein than just rebuilding your cells. When you are on a weight loss program, especially, you need high quality proteins. They will help you build your muscle mass, which in turn will help you burn more calories.

Additionally, proteins consist of Peptide YY, which reduces cravings and also moderates your food consumption. The benefits of proteins last only as long as they are consumed in the required quantity.

While less is bad, more is worse. You need to know how much protein you need.

Ask your nutritionist before you fix a protein requirement for your body. If you do consume too much, it will put a lot of strain on your kidneys.

Health Tip #53 – Good Fats Make You Fit

As absurd as this seems, fats are very important for your body. They are responsible for all the shock absorption in your joints, they help keep your cells in good shape and they are stored to fuel the body in case of any emergency.

But, there are some fats that are healthy and some that are unhealthy.

Fat from sources like fish, olive oil and nuts are good fats as they are packed with essential fatty acids like Omega 3.

In fact, studies at Harvard have revealed that these fats actually help you burn the bad fats in your body.

With healthy fats, you have the advantage of calories. You need to aim to get about 20% of your overall calorie requirement from these sources. They include avocados, nuts, salmon and even some supplements that can be recommended to you by an expert.

Stay away from solid fats like shortening and meat fat., These fats are not really valuable in terms of nutrition and can make up for the bad fats that are stored in your body.

In simple terms, these are the fats that, well, make you fat! So, remember that low fat is not the only choice that you have when it comes to food consumption. Good fats are a good choice.

Health Tip #54 – Curb the Cravings

You can reduce your food cravings with a very simple technique.

All you need to do is get rid of the cue which causes the craving in the first place.

For some people, cravings occur when they are hanging out at the cafeteria with colleagues.

For others, cravings are common when they look at food that is gooey and tempting.

Now, instead of closing your eyes when you see food that is tempting or just ignoring your colleagues when they call you for a quick bite at the cafeteria, here is a simpler thing to do.

Like we discussed before, you need short term and long-term goals. When you feel any craving, focus strongly on your short-term goals. This activates an area of the brain called the prefrontal cortex.

This region will help you cut those cravings instantly. You can also replace the high sugar cravings with healthy alternatives.

This way, you should be able to overcome the cravings eventually.

That is when you will not even be triggered by these common cues that make it hard for most people to focus and eat well.

Health Tip #55 – Avoid Liquid Calories

You can never keep count of your calories when you consume them in the liquid form. Most of us prefer to add a can of soda to every meal.

Well, the thing is, most of these soda pops are just a combination of water and sugar. They are actually saturated with hidden calories. And, with liquids, you never feel like any quantity is too much. Just sip on all day without any count of calories.

Even fruit juice must be limited as it is very high in calories naturally. You must remember that the volume that you consume in liquid form is much higher.

There is very little need to discuss how harmful alcohol is. It is loaded with calories and sugars that do you no good. So, when it comes to consuming calories, make sure you consume them in the solid form and limit them in their liquid form.

Health Tip #56 – Watch Your Habits

There are several common habits that actually have a huge impact on our eating. For instance, if you are used to standing and eating, stop it right now.

Research shows that we eat a lot more food when we are standing.

Also, when we are on a diet, we tend to sneak a bite or two from others' plates. These small bites are those drops of water that make the mighty ocean!

Like we have already seen, eating in front of the TV, eating while working or even eating out regularly are habits that need to be transformed if you are on a serious weight loss program.

Unless you want to give your body more reasons to store up fat and consume more food, you will have to develop healthier habits to make your new eating routine easier to follow.

So, be aware of all the habits that you have developed and change them if required.

Health Tip #57 – Read the Labels

We often get lured by foods with the tags "Low Fat" or "Diet". We all know that there are so many zero sugar and diet colas available in the market.

But, if you were to read their nutritional content, you would be shocked. The amount of sugars, preservatives, carbs and fats that are filled into these foods is critical for you to understand what is going into your body.

So, even if you are picking up the low-fat version of something, read the label. Low fat may mean high sugar sometimes. Until you are convinced that a particular food has the recommended levels of nutrients, you must not pick it up at face value.

Remember, that every product must list the nutritional contents. This is for you, as the consumer, to know what you are actually investing in.

Health Tip #58 – Reduce the Portion That You Cook

A common enemy of any weight loss program is "eating to avoid wasting". For women with families, especially, this is a very common practice. This type of eating leaves you feeling uncomfortable after every meal because you are so stuffed. Of course, it also gives you additional calories that need additional effort to burn.

If you have observed that the quantity of food that you are preparing is always more than you need, try to reduce the quantity. That way, you will eat only what is needed.

If you do have left overs, you can store them and make something else out of it. There are millions of recipes available to help you make the most of all your leftovers.

Just make sure you do not get into the habit of eating to avoid storing food. This is a trap that will definitely hinder the results that you can get from your weight loss program.

Health Tip #59 – A Plan Is Required

If you need to stick to a good eating plan, you have to plan ahead. This means, whenever you go to bed, you need to have all the three meals for the next day planned.

If you need to, you can also make a weekly chart that will help you keep the supplies in stock as well.

What you can do is chart out your entire week's plan and put it up on the refrigerator as a reminder. This way, you know what supplies you need.

For working women, planning ahead is necessary. Eating a planned diet is harder than the regular food that you consume. Those recipes must be on the top of your head and you can do it almost mechanically. But, with new recipes and new foods, it will take a little practice to get used to it. Until that happens, plan ahead.

Health Tip #60 – Do Not Bring It In

You are most likely to consume the forbidden foods if they are easily available. So, the best thing to do would be to just keep it out of your home.

Avoid bringing home any junk. There are times when you have cravings for food while watching a movie or even when you are working late.

That is when you need to have most control. We feel like eating little "fun food" is a great way of rewarding ourselves for all the work that we are putting in.

But you can do nothing about this craving if you don't have the fun foods handy. Then you are forced to adopt the healthier alternative.

As annoying as this seems at first, you can be assured that you will be thankful for developing these habits when you begin to see a slimmer and a fitter you.

That is what you must look forward to than the momentary satisfaction.

Health Tip #61 – Change the Emotional Outlet

For many people, eating is a way of getting hold of their emotions. Have you seen all those chick flicks that advocate eating a bucket of ice cream after you have broken up with someone?

Well, that is just a cliché and a stereotype. You don't need food to suppress negative emotions. That is a psychological process that you can very easily control.

Now, if you are feeling low or unhappy, go for a walk. Do you have a pet at home?

Then, you have the best form of therapy at your disposal. These physical activities and proximity to people you love or even your pets release loads of happy hormones in the body.

That is what you need when you are looking for an emotional outlet.

So, if you know that you only over eat when you are sad or upset, find a new emotional outlet.

Health Tip #62 – Never Buy Food When You Are Hungry

When you are hungry, the natural thing for your body is to crave for foods that are very high in sugar and fat. So, you will be drawn towards these foods.

This is a natural thing and you need not worry about having low will power!

So, when you are hungry, make sure you do not go food shopping as you are likely to pick up the worst foods for yourself.

Instead, try to get a quick snack when before you go out to pick up food.

There is one more trick that you can follow to make sure that you do not shop unnecessarily when it comes to food. Just chew gum as you shop.

This is known to reduce your craving for high sugar and high fat foods almost instantly. You can even chew gum when you are cooking to cleanse your palette and control your appetite.

Health Tip #63 – Divide Your Portions

This is, perhaps, the healthiest way to eat. Your body gets all the nutrition that it needs, in small portions. That way, you are constantly fueled. This avoids any fatigue if you are on a strict weight loss program that involves a good work out.

Additionally, when your body gets its fuel in bits, the storage of fats reduces.

It will make the most of the small portion that you give it and will use it to generate energy. This means calories are also being burnt.

It is also easy on you as your cravings for snacks reduce. Your body also knows that it is going to get foods at regular intervals, which means that you do not have to worry about unwanted fat deposits inside your body.

Health Tip #64 – Keep A Food Journal

A food journal is a great way to ensure success when you are following a diet for weight loss. This helps you keep track of everything that you eat.

That way, you will be able to calculate how much nutrition you managed to get on a daily basis.

No matter what you eat, record the time and the quantity. This even includes a mint or a chocolate.

That way, you can monitor how many unnecessary cups of beverage, how many unwanted calories and fats you are consuming every day.

Cut it down one by one and you will be able to measure your progress soon.

Remember, you are what you eat. Get all your nutrients in the right proportions and you will definitely get all the results that you are aiming for.

The progress is faster when your fitness routine is accompanied by a great diet. All you need is some determination in the beginning. With time, your body will actually lean towards the healthier foods without any conscious effort from your end.

Top Tips to Get Healthy While at Work

When you are at work, it is very easy to lose track of your routine. This is because you are in an environment that is stressful.

You also must be around colleagues who are not leading the healthiest lifestyle. So, you can easily go off track.

When it comes to timing as well, it is very unpredictable. So, you can easily get pulled into the bad habit cycle if you do not take charge and consciously try to get into the groove even at work.

There are many things you can do to stay on your weight loss regime at work. This chapter will discuss in detail how you can overcome those temptations and make your choices matter.

Health Tip #65 – Make A Group

The easiest way to stay focused is to share your goals with your coworkers. You must certainly have many of them in your team who are struggling with weight issues. Make a group with these people and share the goals that you have.

This includes your workout goals and your diet goals. This way, you form your own support system to keep you from cheating or going off track.

What is more that it is fun to have a group of people to share your progress with. When you can share success stories with your group, you will see that the motivation you get is instantaneous.

Health Tip #66 – Have Water Bottles Handy

It is common to feel really hungry when you are working for several hours at a stretch. So, keep a reusable water bottle on your table.

That way, you can take a sip every time you have the urge to snack unnecessarily. Yes, you will have a dedicated snack time when you can refuel yourself.

But, when it comes to the cravings in between, water is a great way to ward them off.

In addition to that, water will keep you hydrated at all times. This makes you less lethargic and more focused towards your work. Water also helps dissolve fats that are stored in your body. So, water at the work place is a lifesaver.

Health Tip #67 – Eat with People

Most of us tend to eat before the computer screen. This accounts for mindless eat. It is just as good as eating in front of a TV. We discussed the weight related issues that you may develop because of that.

Instead, you could choose to eat with your colleagues. Talking to them will also reduce the amount of food that you eat as you tend to take breaks.

Research shows that our brain takes 20 minutes to register the fact that the stomach is full. So, people who gulp their food tend to feel hungry for longer and also tend to eat more food.

But, if you rest your cutlery for some chitchat and then get on with your eating, you will definitely eat lesser. Of course, good company is also a great way to bust the stress.

Health Tip #68 – Keep Your Toothbrush with You

Brushing your teeth after your meals and snacks is a great way to avoid fueling your body with unwanted calories.

You see, we always tend to pick a candy from the neighbor's bowl to feel fresh and energized after a meal.

Otherwise, you may feel drowsy and lethargic. But, when you brush your teeth, you will instantly feel energized.

In addition to that, once your palette is cleansed, your craving for certain kinds of foods also reduces instantly.

When you go to work, keep your tooth brush handy. If you feel like that is a lot of work, you may also try a mouthwash immediately after you eat for the same effect.

The only thing you need to remember is that mint and candy is loaded with sugars that we are trying to avoid for quick weight loss and toning.

Health Tip #69 – Set Reminders

Don't restrict the reminders on your computer and your phone to work related things. You can also set reminders for your own personal weigh loss program.

You can set reminders for various things like walking around the office, stretching, taking your supplements or even eating your snacks.

If you need reminders to watch your eating habits, you can work with them.

For instance, if you have a snack break at 4pm, your reminder can say "Choose an apple instead of pastries, you just lost 400 grams".

These reminders keep you in touch with the progress that you have made and will also tell you what your priorities are.

Health Tip #70 – Watch Those Shoes

The most common excuse given by women for walking in the office is that their shoes are uncomfortable.

Do you know that just by walking around the office, you can burn as many calories as you need to in a day?

So, even if you have to ditch the regular cardio routine, this will come handy.

In addition to that, more physical activity means less fat and fewer calories. That is why you must make sure that the shoes you wear to work are comfortable.

It is one of the silliest excuses that you can come up with to avoid walking around. If required, keep a change of shoes in your office.

Wear the uncomfortable glamorous ones only when you have to meet clients or, perhaps, go to certain events. At all other times, get comfortable and get moving!

Health Tip #71 – Avoid Instant Messaging

Instant messaging is the reason for all the laziness in the office set up. In the earlier days, you had to walk up to the next cabin to deliver a message.

That is why people were healthier and also had better focus on the work that they were doing. It is so easy to lose focus when you are seated in one place all day, isn't it?

Instead, you could walk over to your colleague and talk, just like the good old days. This will keep you active and will also help you cut those calories faster.

Instant messaging is good for emergency memos. But, if you just want to share some gossip or talk generally, do it in person. You will have some reason to walk around.

And who does not look forward to small talk in office. So, that gives you motivation as well!

Health Tip #72 – Swiss Balls Are Great

We all have really comfortable chairs at work. These chairs are designed ergonomically to keep our back supported and also ensure the right posture.

While it is recommended that you use these chairs for most part of the day, it would do you great good to deviate for an hour or so each day.

Just keep a Swiss ball in your office. For an hour every day, replace your chair with it.

When you are working while you are sitting on the Swiss ball, your core muscles are fully engaged. Now, that is a great way to get rid of that tummy fat that you have been struggling with for the longest time now.

It also strengthens your back and core and gives you better posture for everything else that you do throughout the day.

Health Tip #73 – Keep the Coffee Black

Black coffee is less fattening and is also more energizing. Adding milk to it makes it unhealthier that it already is. Now, if you must drink coffee, cut the sugar out.

You may not be able to do this immediately. But you can gradually reduce the amount of sugar that you add to your coffee. This is an effective way to watch the calories that get into your body. At your workplace, coffee is the biggest source of unwanted sugars.

If possible, replace coffee with green tea. While it is a myth that green tea alone can help you lose weight, it is true that green tea is loaded with several antioxidants. So, this cleanses your system and gives you a good instant detox.

That way, all the processes that you have engaged in your body to result in weight loss will be catalyzed by the green tea.

You will also have the psychological satisfaction of having a hot beverage when you need it. That will keep you focused at work as well.

Health Tip #74 – Carry Your Lunch

We get into several poor eating habits primarily because we need to eat out when at work.

If you are working late someday, plan ahead like we discussed before and carry all the meals and snacks that you require till you get home.

This will certainly prevent loading up on unwanted sugars and fats. You will also be able to watch the portion that you are consuming.

There is no temptation when you do this because, let's face it, you do not want to waste all the food that you have cooked yourself. So, you will be able to make healthier eating choices.

Health Tip #75 – Protein-Rich Snacks

Snacks that are rich in proteins are very good for you. They will curb hunger and they will give you additional benefits like increased muscle mass.

You can keep a protein bar, nuts or even a few boiled eggs with you for that post lunch hunger. With these natural protein sources, you also have other nutrients like Omega 3 that will be added to your system.

Protein rich snacks are good even when you are feeling tired as they will give you instantaneous energy as well. So, carry something in your handbag or in your drawer at all times.

Health Tip #76 – Healthier Dessert Options

If you have coworkers who carry big desserts to work, it is easy to give in to the craving. Instead, what you can do is carry your own healthier dessert option. That way, you can still enjoy the complete meal without feeling left out.

Some of the best options are granola bars, yoghurt and fruits or just a nice fruit salad.

They will make up for the sugar cravings while loading your body up with several other nutrients that it requires keeping up with your rigorous weight loss regime.

Health Tip #77 – Plan Workouts

When you head back home, the last thing you want to do it leave again for a workout. People who plan to get home and then get to the gym are the ones who miss their sessions the most.

If you are working out at home, it is best to do it before you head out to the office, as you are fresher.

On the other hand, if you plan to attend a gym or a group class plan for it when you are coming home from the office or when you are getting to the office from your home. This is likely to improve your attendance.

You see, staying focused at work does not demand too much work. The only thing you need is a little bit of conscious discipline in the initial days.

After you see the slightest results, these habits and practices will become second skin. The positive results will make you greedy for better. And, this type of greed is completely acceptable as it puts you on a lifelong path of health and fitness.

Others who are considering purchasing this book would love to know what you think. If you could spare a few seconds, they would greatly appreciate reading an honest review from you. Simply visit the page on Amazon.com.

Top Tips to Stay Healthy at Home

The maximum number of distractions for any workout routine exists at home. This is where you want to just put your feet up and enjoy some time for yourself. You do not want to be told what you can eat and what you need to do for a better body.

This is also the primary reason why you fail most often when you get back home. No matter how determined you are after talking to your fitness group that can of soda in the refrigerator does tempt you.

So, if you want to keep the regime on 24X7 what you must do is watch your habits when you are home. If you can overcome bad habits at home, then you will be able to continue this just about anywhere in the world.

This section will give you tips that will ensure faster weight loss and toning by improving your habits in the comfort of your home.

Health Tip #78 – The 80/20 Rule

It is a terrible feeling to be in control at all times. This is especially true when you are at home. You need some time to chill out and take a break. When you are being too rigid or too stuck on ideas, you tend to feel stressed.

So, keep the 80/20 rule in mind. This means your keep the discipline 80% and leave 20% room to have fun. That way you will never miss out on family fun nights!

Health Tip #79 – Keep the Fridge Stocked

The fridge can make or break your diet. If it is not stocked with the right foods, there is a definite chance that you will binge on something unhealthy.

So, make it a point to go and shop for food at least once a week.

Draw up a weekly plan to help you shop better. You can make a list of all the foods that you need to complete your meals and to make up for your snacks.

When this is done, you do not have to hold yourself back from reaching out into your refrigerator.

Health Tip #80 – Send Your Food Journal to Someone

Pick a family member or a friend to send the food journal to. Do this on a daily basis via an email.

Remember to be honest as this is only for your good. You can type the journal out in the form of an email and send it to a family member every night.

This will give you a sense of accountability and the chances of cheating will reduce considerably.

If you have someone who already has the healthy gig going on, choose him or her as the one you want to mail the journal to. That will give you more reason to be careful about what you eat.

Health Tip #81 – Keep A Notice Board

In the kitchen, keep a notice board or even a chalkboard. Put up your goals on this board and develop the habit of putting up a motivational saying on it every day.

When you move around the kitchen, having this board in sight will remind you of your priorities and will keep you focused on what you need to do to keep the weight loss plan going.

The reason I tell you to choose the kitchen is that it is the central part of the house and you are likely to visit this space most often.

Health Tip #82 – Pictures on The Fridge

Take a picture of yours on a weekly basis and put it up on the refrigerator. When you take a new picture, put the old one in a jar.

After a month, you can compare the first and the last picture to see the difference.

These picture jars are very motivating because a disciplined diet and weight loss plan is bound to give you the results that you want.

It will give you the push that you need to keep the transformation going until you have a picture of your dream body up on the fridge.

Health Tip #83 – Overcome Boredom

The easiest way to overcome boredom is to cuddle up before the TV with a bag of chips or a bucket of ice cream. Instead, you must find ways to overcome boredom that do not involve food.

This includes things like walking, going out into the garden, picking fruits, reading or even something more beneficial like yoga.

When you can overcome boredom, you automatically reduce binging on junk foods. Now, that is precisely what you need to keep yourself in control even when you are at home.

In simpler terms, find a hobby and stick to it to improve the weight loss process.

Health Tip #84 – Sleep Well

When you do not have enough sleep, your body is under stress. This means that the levels of stress hormones increase, too. With this comes fat storage.

Sleeping also helps you burn a lot of calories as your system is in overdrive, repairing muscles and tissues. This is when maximum recovery happens.

You also have more energy and more motivation when you are well rested.

Weight loss is directly associated with sleep as several factors like metabolism and nutrition uptake come into play with sleep. So, the best way to continue the process at home is to sleep well.

Health Tip #85 – Drink Water

You need to drink water always. But you need to do this even more when you are at home. At home, you need this reminder simply because you have other alternatives like soda to distract you.

When you are in the state of relaxing, your body does not give you signals like thirst. So, you don't know that you need water. Therefore, keep yourself consciously hydrated when you are at home.

This also keeps your appetite in check and reduces untimely food cravings.

Health Tip #86 – Wear the Right Clothes

Ladies, avoid wearing baggy clothes at home. Yes, this does count as a very important weight loss tip. With baggy clothes, you cannot see the flabs that you want to get rid of.

This means that the visual cue that makes you want to work out and lose weight is absent. That is why it is that much easier to slack off at home.

During the day, wear clothes that fit you properly so you can see the problem areas.

This will keep you on your toes and will prevent the development of lazy habits and bad habits over the weekend.

With this very simple practice, you will notice that you have the determination even when you are at home.

Health Tip #87 – Always Have Fruits & Vegetables at Hand

Having to cut up carrots into sticks just before your favorite show makes you reach out for a packed snack.

So, if you know that you are going to be spending time at home, cut up those veggies and fruits beforehand. That way, you have no excuse to go for the shortcuts, namely the processed foods.

It is easier to choose a healthy snack when it is readily available.

Most often the mental image of scarping and cutting up the veggies and then cleaning it up can demotivate you more than you think.

Health Tip #88 – Make A Vision Chart

A vision chart is a must have for all the busy ladies who need constant reminders.

Put up your goals with images to keep the cues coming. This is a great way to stay on track even when you feel like chucking it all.

Place the vision chart in places that you look at the most. This could be the door of your cupboard, your fridge or even the switchboard closest to the door.

You will constantly look at the vision board when you are at home. Your brain receives the message on a sub conscious level, making it easier for you to stay on track.

Health Tip #89 – Stick on Comments

Place stick on comments on various things. This includes you tub of ice cream, the snack counter, the TV remote etc.

Small notes like "Eat this now, regret later"; "Remember, how hard you worked to get here?"; "Go, get some exercise" can really help you stay on your toes when you are home.

Yes, you can tell yourself this but the voices in your head can argue and make you weak.

But visual cues will never fail to give you that constant reminder that you need to keep the plan going.

Health Tip #90 – Use Smaller Plates

Research shows that reducing the size of your plate will automatically reduce the food portions. This is because we always think that we have enough to eat when the plate is full.

So, logically, a smaller plate fills up faster than a bigger one. Your brain tells you that you have had a plate full of food and hence you must be full.

These exercises prove that so many eating habits that we cultivate are purely psychological.

If you can put mind over matter, you can really accomplish anything that you want to. Actually, weight loss is completely in control of your mind.

Health Tip #91 – Drink A Glass of Red Wine

Yes, alcohol contains a lot of calories. This is when we compare the risk and the benefit. When it comes to red wine, the benefits are so many that you are permitted one glass a day. Now, I can imagine that this is where you are saying, "I love losing weight!"

Red wine contains resveratrol, which is a great anti-oxidant. It helps release the fat that is stored in your body. But remember, that you can only have a small glass of wine for the benefits. That is roughly about 125 ml and not more.

For those of you who do not prefer wine, blueberries, pomegranate and cranberries are great sources of resveratrol for your body.

Health Tip #92 – Please Don't Make This MISTAKE

One of the first things you need to pay attention to when you want a lean and sexy body is your nutrition. It does not matter how much you work out and tone if you are eating the wrong kinds of food or eating improperly.

The first thing that you should do for a lean body is to eat breakfast.

While many people will cut breakfast out because they think it will save them on calories, it could actually be harming your weight loss goals.

There have been many studies done that show that eating a healthy breakfast every morning is able to help you lose weight while skipping out could make you gain back more weight.

This is thought to be because you will be more likely to overeat in the evening if you missed out on breakfast.

You also need to make your breakfast smart; choosing a sugar treat like a donut or a small granola bar will not help you out. Choose a balanced breakfast for the best results.

Health Tip #93 – How to Listen to Your Body

Do not worry about when you think it is time to eat. Many people feel that they need to eat at a certain time because that is the norm, but if you are not hungry, you are feeding your body more nutrients than it needs.

Only eat when you get the right cues from the body and you will be amazed at how lean you can get form the weight loss. If it is lunch time and you do not feel hungry, do not eat.

Wait until your body decides that it is hungry and then you can eat the meal that works for that part of the day.

This is something that might be a little difficult to get used to in the beginning. Your body is used to eating at certain times and eating certain amounts so it might feel like it is hungry all of the time.

You might want to consider doing a detox or other diet that is similar for a couple of days to get the body back on track.

After some practice, you will be able to get the hunger cues back on track and help your body to just eat when it is hungry.

Health Tip #94 – The #1 MISTAKE Women Make on Diets

While skipping meals might seem like a good way to cut out the calories and get more weight loss, it usually does not work this way for most people. Instead of cutting the calories, most people will end up eating more of them later on.

When you eat in a healthy way and get in the meals that you need rather than skipping them, you are promoting healthier choices later on. Remember that you need to eat meals that are healthy and wholesome at regular intervals throughout the day as well as some snacks.

While you should only eat when you are feeling hungry, these regular meals can help to prevent overeating later on in the day and can make sure that your metabolism stays going strong.

Health Tip #95 – The Optimal Way to Consume Protein

If you want to get that lean look, you might want to consider going vegetarian. Studies have shown that cutting out the meat that is in your diet can lead to a leaner look.

While meat might have a ton of protein in it, there is also the issue with having a lot of calories and cholesterol inside, especially when it comes to the size portions that most Americans eat.

Protein is still important to your diet though.

You can still get enough of the protein that your body needs simply by eating it through plant sources.

Of course, you do not have to go on a vegetarian diet in order to get the lean look that you are going for. It is possible to get that lean look, although vegetarians are more likely to have it.

If you choose to not go on a vegetarian diet, you should still watch for portion control on the meats that you are eating.

Keep the portions small and try to choose some lean options such as turkey and chicken as well as fish rather than going with unhealthier options such as beef.

Health Tip #96 – A Quick Fix with MANY Benefits

Sugars are a horrible thing to eat if you are looking to lose weight and get that lean and sexy body.

A diet that has a low amount of added sugars is one that has fewer calories, especially the ones that are empty and do not add any benefits to the body.

A report that come through the Centers for Disease Control and Prevention in 2013 defined the added sugars as those that are added into prepared and processed foods such as ice cream, jam, cakes and breads.

You can find this added sugar in many of the foods you eat and avoiding it can sometimes be difficult. Being diligent and watching what you eat can make a lot of differences.

This is the most difficult thing that most people have to do when they are trying to go on any diet, much less get the lean and sexy look.

You will have to cut out on many of the foods that you love and might have cravings for. Things like candy, soda (even diet soda), donuts, pastries, cake, and so much more will need to be cut out of the diet.

This may be hard, but just think of how great the rewards are going to be when you are done.

Health Tip #97 – How to Eat More Vegetables the EASY Way

Vegetables are going to be your new best friend on this journey. They are going to provide you with a lot of the nutrition that you need with very low calories so that you can get the best of both worlds. Try to add some vegetables into all of your meals and snacks in order to get the fiber and other nutrients you need in order to lose some weight.

There are a lot of ways that you will be able to add in vegetables. You could just add them in on the side of your meal and have a good serving of it each time.

You could mix it into a casserole or other dish that you are eating to get them. There are a lot of snacks that you can eat that will have vegetables as part of the dish so that you can get the nutrients.

You should aim for about 5 to 6 servings of the vegetables in order to get the best results. The more vegetables you can get, the better you will feel, the fuller you will get, and the easier it will be to lose the weight that you would like.

Health Tip #98 – Which Grains Actually Matter

Yes, there are some options that are less than the 100%, but you should always stick with the best.

The whole grain variety is the one that will give you the most nutrients, help you to feel fuller for longer, and prevents you from gaining weight.

The other versions will pretty much do the opposite. You want to feed your body the very best when it comes to losing weight and getting a lean body. 100% grains are the ones you need to concentrate on in order to give your body the best.

There are a lot of grains that you will need to avoid if you would like to get healthy. Do not eat pastas, pizzas, donuts, and other sweets that have been processed.

These really are just full of sugars that are not good for you and can make it difficult to lose the weight that you would like.

Choose the healthier whole wheat and whole grain versions of these that you would normally eat in order to get the best nutrition and health for your calories.

Health Tip #99 – Use Smaller Containers

You should get into the habit of using containers that are smaller. Often the size of container you pick will dictate how much food you will put into the thing.

When you have more food in front of you, it is much easier to put it all in your mouth, even when you are not hungry or you know that you should not eat the extra food.

Pick out a container that is smaller and only fill it up a little bit. You will consume fewer calories and see the weight melt off.

A good way to do this is to just throw away all of the old big containers that you have at home. You are no longer going to need them so there is no point in them being there.

Just keep the smaller containers so that you are not tempted to take on bigger meals or portions. Use the container to plan out your meals in order to keep calories low and nutrition high.

Health Tip #100 – How You Should NOT Cut Calories

While you might be doing a great job with counting calories and making sure that you are taking in the right nutrition and calorie amounts to lose weight, it is still possible to not lose any weight.

This is because you might be drinking the calories that you are consuming.

Think about those sodas, coffees, smoothies, and other specialty drinks that you are taking in. Unless you are drinking water, you are adding more calories into your day and this can often add up pretty quickly in some drinks.

It is better to spend your time drinking water and a little bit of herbal tea in order to keep the calories down and just consuming healthy foods with nutrients.

If you must, limit your coffee to one cup a day and cut out the cream and sugar.

It is best if you are able to just limit your drink content just to water and herbal tea. While it is fine to have some milk and some juice without added sugar, but water is the best option because it will keep you hydrated without all of the extra calories.

You should limit your consumption of alcohol and sodas, even the diet kind, because they are not healthy and they will just dehydrate you a lot more.

Health Tip #101 – Balanced Meals Are Important

Make sure that the meals you are consuming are balanced and healthy. You should have all of the major food groups present on your plate and a lot of color is often recommended.

Make sure the fruits and veggies are there as well as some kind of dairy and a protein source.

Eating this balanced meal can help you to feel fuller for longer and prevents you from overeating or making bad health decisions later on.

Each meal that you create should be as balanced as possible and your snacks should not be full of chips and ice cream. While it is fine to splurge on occasion if you really can't help it, you should make sure to only do this when necessary.

Also, avoid the fast food restaurants, they are not going to provide you with the good health that you need and there is no balance whatsoever in the food outside of having tons of calories, fats, and other things that are bad for you.

Choose foods that are healthy and which will help you to get closer to your own goals. Try to include a lean protein source, some whole wheat, some dairy perhaps in the form of a glass of milk, and plenty of fruits and vegetables.

There are also plenty of snacks you can choose from that include fresh fruits and vegetables to keep you healthy.

Proper nutrition is imperative if you want to get the healthy and lean body that matches the celebrities. You can work out all that you would like and put as much effort into it as you can and you might see some results, but the final look that you are going for is not going to happen until you are able to get in the right nutrition.

The hints that are given in this chapter should help to lead you in the right direction to looking and feeling your very best. Keep them in mind each and every time that you plan out a meal.

Health Tip #102 – Don't Forget the Goal

Write it in big letters, print it out, call up a friend and do whatever you have to in order to announce that you are going to be losing weight and getting the body that you have always wanted.

The more you announce the news, the more likely you will get up and get out there to do the work.

This is because you have basically made a promise not just to yourself but to others around you and you will feel like they are holding you accountable.

Health Tip #103 – You NEED This for Real Success

You will never be able to reach your goal without some support on hand. Find someone who can keep you motivated through a quick call or a message to let you know that they are proud of what you have accomplished.

Or even better, find someone who will go out there and get the exercise done with you.

This support group is to be there for you through it all and can keep you going even when you are ready to quit.

Health Tip #104 – If You Can Start Out Like This, You Can Get Healthy FASTER

Sometimes you are having difficulties with getting started because the task is just too big in your head. You might start out with the task that is about losing all of the weight and if there is quite a bit to lose, this can be daunting.

Think about the first few pounds that you want to lose and concentrate just on that.

The same goes for your workouts; you do not have to start out with doing intense workouts a few times a week but instead can do some small ones to start and slowly build up.

Health Tip #105 – A Great Tip to Help YOU Stick to Your Health Plan

You are never going to reach your fitness goals if you do not stick with it. Even if it is hard and you would rather be doing something else, just give it the time that it needs.

Often half the battle is getting your shoes on and getting to the gym. Once you are able to get that far, you will at least be able to convince yourself to get a good workout done since you are already there.

Health Tip #106 – You Cannot Be Negative

Any time that you have a negative thought about the progress that you are making, you need to squash it right away. Only positive thoughts are allowed in this game and that is the only way that you will succeed.

Just keeping thinking that you will be able to do it and that you will get through it rather than this is hard and I will never be able to finish it.

Health Tip #107 – How to Set Real Goals That WORK

You should always have some kind of goals in place so that you are able to know when you are getting something accomplished or not.

Especially if you just go to the gym each day without any idea of what you are doing or if you are actually doing something.

When you have a goal in place, you can tell if you are heading in the right direction or if you need to work harder in order to get it all accomplished.

Make sure that the goals you are going for are realistic and that you will actually be able to accomplish them with a little hard work.

Health Tip #108 – Please Avoid Doing This to Yourself

It is easy to get on your own case if you miss out on a workout or if you do not do as well as you would like on something. Things happen and life gets in the way and sometimes things do not go the way that you would like them to.

If you berate yourself and make yourself feel like you are not doing a good job, it can be difficult to get the motivation to get back to work.

On those days that you are not able to do a good job or not make it to the gym, just remember that you can go another day and promise that you will just work harder the next time to make up.

Health Tip #109 – A Cool Gadget to Help You

Yes, these might seem a little bit cheesy and like something that would be a waste of your time, but you would be amazed at how much more you will be able to work out when you have these.

You should try some that will keep track of your heart rate, steps, and more so that you are able to keep track of the progress as you go. Try to keep up with the results of your good days and find out how well you will be able to do each day.

Health Tip #110 – Set Real Rewards

Every time that you reach a goal that you have set, you should find a good treat that will make you feel good.

You should make sure that it does not have something to do with eating or food because you are trying to lose weight.

But you also want to make sure that you are picking a reward that is going to keep you motivated to keep on working hard.

These are just a few of the things that you can do in order to stay motivated and get yourself to the gym when you need to. Make sure to use as many as you can in order to get the best results each and every time.

Health Tip #111 – Limit Your Workouts

Many people feel that they need to spend an hour or more at the gym. This is just not true as long as you do a high interval and intense workout instead.

Once you go above the 40-minute market, you just are not getting the great workout that you were for the beginning because you need to decrease the intensity in order to keep up.

Doing a shorter really intense program can cause more weight loss and make you feel that your workout was really worth it.

Health Tip #112 – HIIT is the KEY to Weight Loss

These are actually much more effective than the longer workouts that you are used to. Instead of spending so much time at the gym, you will just spend a short amount of time getting a great workout in.

These kinds of exercises are going to push you to the max and will take all that you got, if they are working properly. But the time limit will be about 30 minutes or so compared to an hour or more working out at your normal pace.

You also have the added benefit of being healthier; high intensity workouts are better for the heart and overall health compared to other options.

Health Tip #113 – Why You're Missing Out If You Don't Lift

It is common practice at the gym for someone to contract up the muscle going slowly and then they will release the muscle quickly.

If you want to do really get a good workout, you should make sure that you are lifting slowly in each direction in order to get the move maximized.

You might want to start adding on a little more weight, up to what you are comfortable in, to get started. This is going to work the muscles much harder and make you get an amazing workout.

Health Tip #114 – Compounding Exercises

Why spend all of that time at the gym just working on one muscle group at a time?

Doesn't this seem like a big waste of your time and completely inefficient?

It is possible to compound the workouts that you are doing in order to get more than one muscle group to be worked out at the same time.

There are even a few workouts that you can do that will get the whole body worked out in just a few steps.

Try to do these as much as possible; not only will they give you a better workout, but it is also going to help in real life application since you use more than one muscle to get things done in day to day life.

Health Tip #115 – When You Lift, Do This

Some people will work out a muscle group for a few reps, stop, and then go and do it a few times.

A better idea is to just keep lifting a weight until you are not able to continue doing it with the proper form.

Once you reach this point, which is going to vary depending on how good of shape you are in for how many you can do, you are done with that workout.

Health Tip #116 – Pick Your Workouts on Purpose

If you want to keep going with the workouts that you are doing, you need to pick one that you really enjoy. Otherwise you will become bored and not want to keep up with the process.

Pick a good weight lifting and a good cardio workout and even find ways to combine the two so that you are getting the most efficient workout each and every time.

There are a lot of choices that you can go with such as rowing, Stairmaster, hiking, biking, swimming, running, and even some home videos.

The choice is not as important as you having fun with doing the workout and keeping up with it for the long term.

Health Tip #117 – Variety Is Crucial

It can be easy to stick with just one workout all of the time. You might be used to doing it or you think that you should just be concentrating on certain areas in order to get the results, but you really need to mix it up every once in a while.

First, this mixing up is going to make sure that the workout stays fun and exciting because it helps you to stay motivated at doing the workout and can even make you work out harder.

Second, if you are doing the same work out all of the time your body is going to become efficient with dealing with it and you will not be able to get the same results that you are looking for.

Health Tip #118 – Try Circuit Training for Health Benefits

Circuits are a great way to get in your good workout. These are nice in several ways.

First, you are allowing the body to get a break between the exercises that you are doing. If you keep working out the same muscles or muscle groups without giving them the break that they need, you will find that the muscle will get worn out and might be led to an injury.

This is not good for the body and can prevent you from continuing the workout in the future. With circuit training, you will be alternating between several different activities which makes it easier to give your muscles the rest that they need.

In addition, since you are doing a variety of activities, you will be able to work out a variety of body parts in a smaller amount of time. It is a win win for your body and can also be a lot of fun.

Getting a good all-around workout is critical if you are looking to lose weight and get in shape.

That slim and sexy body does not happen on its own and you need to make sure that you are doing a good workout that will get the heart running, the muscles burning, and your body ready to get toned and lean.

Health Tip #119 – Please Don't Forget This Tip

Drinking plenty of water is important if you want to have a slim and sexy body. It is hard to stay fit if you are not giving your body the water that it needs.

Workouts will become more difficult, you will feel light headed and the body is just not going to work as efficiently as it did in the past.

Plus, when you drink plenty of water you are able to fill up your stomach much faster and could avoid many of the snacking cravings that you usually do. This can help you to lose weight overall.

This chapter is going to spend some time going over the importance of drinking plenty of water and tips on how to get more water into your daily routine.

Health Tip #120 – Your "Go To" In the Morning

Early in the morning, you might be antsy about waiting for the coffee or the hot tea to brew.

You love the first sip of coffee and how it feels when it is going down your throat in order to wake you up.

But that darn waiting time can be such a pain. While you are waiting, you can have a nice glass of water to help prepare.

Add some herbal tea and a little bit of lemon if you would like or just enjoy the warm glass of water on its own. This is a great way to stay warm and cozy, get the water that your body needs every day, and to make the wait until the coffee comes more enjoyable.

Health Tip #121 – An Important Investment with Big Benefits

If you are going to make the commitment to drink more water, get a bottle that can make it more fun. There have been surveys done that show people who are able to have a fun and interesting bottle are more likely to drink out of it.

Go to the store and spend some money on a nice one that you can use that is heavy duty and ready to go wherever the day takes you.

You could even slap some stickers or other things on the bottle if you are not able to find one that is exactly what you would like. Take it around wherever you go during the day and drink any time that you think about it.

The second the bottle gets empty, go and fill it up again so you can keep getting hydrated. Never let your body get thirsty or you have already begun getting dehydrated.

Health Tip #122 – A Small Tip with Big Impacts

Thinking about taking big gulps of water in order to get the recommended eight glasses can be daunting. That just seems like a lot of work to get done when you have to do it all at once.

But when you are able to split up the work and do it little at a time, it can become a whole lot easier. All you will need to do is put a straw into the cup and then just sip a little bit at a time.

Sip a little bit while waiting on line for someone, while checking your emails, at a meeting, or just when you are taking a break from other work.

You will be surprised at how much more water you are able to consume just by putting in a straw and soon it will be all gone.

In fact, studies of shown that people are more likely to drink more water each day if they are able to do it through a straw rather than through other means.

Health Tip #123 – Vitamin Water

If you are having trouble with getting in the vitamins that you need to stay strong or you just do not like the taste of water that much, consider making your own vitamin water.

There are a variety of store brands that are available which can help you just make some on the go or you can make your own.

Many of these recipes are going to have some added flavoring so you will be able to add in a little bit of taste to your drink rather than just drinking old boring water.

Just be careful with the types you buy at the store or that you make.

It is not going to do any good for your nutrition if you are consuming a ton of sugar in these packets of vitamin water.

Even when you are making the juices on your own, you should make sure that you are not accidentally adding in more sugar than is necessary.

Health Tip #124 – Health Benefits of Filtered Water

One of the biggest reasons that people will not consume enough water is that they just do not like or can't stand the taste. This is because many times the water in cities and from the well just tastes horrible.

There is an easy way to fix this problem. Just go to the store and pick out one of the filters that are available. There are many different choices that you can make when it comes to filters.

Some will hook right on your faucet and you can switch it on and off in order to get clean drinking water or so that you can regular water for cooking and cleaning. Or you can get one of the pitcher options.

This will allow you to fill up the pitcher and then keep the water cool in the fridge or on the counter to drink whenever you wish.

This will allow you to easily clean out the water and get it to taste great so you can enjoy it again.

Health Tip #125 – How Habit Stacking Can Help You

There are things you do throughout the day that have become kind of habits. Make sure to pair up water with them in order to get the hydration that your body needs.

For example, you can choose to have a cup of water with each meal and snack that you take in. If you like to take a long bath a few times a week, have a glass of water while you are doing that.

While you are working out, make sure to keep a bottle of water right next to you and refill it every time that you need to. Just make sure that you keep some water near you at all times. The more available the water is the more likely that you will take a drink and stay as hydrated as you can.

Health Tip #126 – Track Water Consumption

You might be surprised at how little water you are taking in each day. It is easy to get distracted by other things and not get the water that you need into your body.

What's even worse, many people will drink other things, like sodas and alcohol, that not only prevent you from drinking enough water, they also can dehydrate out your body like crazy. All of this is going to combine to make you dehydrated and not suitable for getting a good workout or losing the weight that you want.

When you track the consumption that you are taking in, it is easier to find out if you are doing a good job or if you need to work harder.

Spend a week tracking how much liquids you take in whether it is from milk, juice, water, soda, or some other source. You should be able to get a good idea of the consumption that you are dealing with.

You might not realize how much you are consuming of the bad liquids compared to the good liquids. Then you can work from there and try to find ways that you will be able to take in more water and limit the other kinds of liquids.

While it is fine to get some other liquids on occasion, you should limit it to mostly water with a little bit of milk for dairy and limited amounts of juice without added sugar.

Health Tip #127 – Water Has Bigger Benefits Than Anything Else – Make It a Goal

You should start out with making a goal on how much water you would like to consume each day.

This can make it easier to track what you are doing and can help you to get more. Start the first week by taking in an extra glass each day, and then two, and then three.

Keep going with this until you have made it to at least the 8 recommended glasses of water for the day or more if you are really working out hard.

This goal can help you to have an end point in mind where you will be able to work hard and know whether you are getting to that point or not.

Health Tip #128 – Competitions Make It Exciting

Humans like to compete with each other and there is no better way to make sure that you are getting the water that you need. It can become more of a game rather than a chore that you have to get done.

Find a coworker, friend or someone in your family who is looking to get more water into their routine or who would at least be able to do the process with you.

Both of you can have a competition together in order to see who will be able to either drink the most amount of water in the whole week or who is able to reach their goals the most during the week.

You can even set up a prize for the person who is able to do the best over a certain amount of time or just have some fun with each other without prizes.

It is all up to you the way that you would like to get it done. Just make sure that both of you are having fun while getting the water that you need into your day.

Health Tip #129 – Thirsty or Hungry?

One reason that people will eat more calories than they need is because they are eating when they are actually hungry. This is a common problem that a lot of people have because their bodies will send out the feelings of hunger rather than of thirst.

When you feel hungry, your first thought is to eat something rather than to take something to drink.

Of course, this is not the best idea to do when you just finished eating, but most people do not think about it and will just continue eating even when they might not be that hungry.

This can add in more calories and make it difficult to get the slim body that you are looking for.

If you have just eaten, you should not continue to eat when you feel the pains of hunger. You are most likely just thirsty. Drink a cup of cold water and then wait a few minutes.

For the most part, this is going to be enough to fill up the hunger pains and you will not take in more calories than you need. If this does not work and you still feel some hunger, go ahead and eat a little bit more.

You can also do this all throughout the day to make sure that you are only eating when you are hungry rather than eating when your body is actually thirsty.

These are some of the simple tips that you can use in order to get some more water into your diet.

This can sometimes be difficult to do at first because most people think that they are getting more water in to the diet than they actually are.

When they find out how little they are taking in, they are amazed and feel that 8 cups is almost impossible.

But if you follow just a few of these tips, getting the required amount of water will be simple and easy.

Try a few of these out today to start out your new routine.

Health Tip #130 – The Benefits of a Regular Bed Time

You should make sure that you are going to bed at the same time each night. You can pick the time, but make sure that it is at close to the same time each night.

Do not go down early throughout the week and then stay up late on the weekends because this simple habit could completely throw of the sleep schedule that you have.

Choose sometime when you are going to be tired naturally rather than just forcing yourself to go to sleep because you think it is time and then wasting time tossing and turning in bed.

If a later bed time is good for you, then that is fine as long as you make sure to figure out one that will work most nights of the week. Try not to mix it all up so that you can get into a regular cycle.

If something comes up and you need to switch around your schedule, you should do it slowly and not all at once or you could really make it difficult.

Try to just stay up 15 minutes later or earlier each day until you finally make it to the new time that you want to set up. Once you have that new time, try to keep it regular for the best results.

Health Tip #131 – Wake Up Routine

Just like with going to bed at the same time each night, you need to get into a routine of waking up at the same time each day.

If you are doing this right and getting the sleep that you need, then you should be able to wake up without an alarm clock naturally.

For those who need an alarm clock, you might need to find an earlier bedtime to get into the right groove of what needs to be done Try to keep this all organized and get up at the same time each day, even on the weekend.

Health Tip #132 – When You Can, Take A Nap

Sometimes it is hard to get the regular sleep time that you need each day.

If you have kids you might have to get up a few times in the night to take care of them, you might have had some trouble staying asleep a few nights, or you had some trouble going to bed because of work or other obligations to take care of.

These things can make it difficult in order to get the sleep that you need.

One solution to this is to take a nap throughout the day. You can take a nap sometime during the day in order to make up for the lost time rather than sleeping later in the day.

This is better because you will not have ruined your schedule like you would if you are staying in bed late, but you will still be able to catch up on the sleep that you are feeling.

You will need to be smart about the sleep that you are getting. If you do it incorrectly, you will find that insomnia will be your friend at night and it could really throw off the sleep schedule that you are on.

Try to keep the napping down to thirty minutes and if you find that insomnia shows up when you take naps, cut them out completely.

Health Tip #133 – How to Fight Sleepy Feelings

Many people will find that they get really drowsy after they get to supper time and eat a good meal.

If you do feel that you are getting sleepy and you still have a few hours before it is time to go to bed, it is important to get up and go do something that can stimulate you at least a little bit.

This can help you to not fall asleep before it is time. You can do the dishes, call a friend and have a good conversation, or even just clean a room. Do not do too much work because you might get the adrenaline running and you will not be able to fall asleep later.

Health Tip #134 – Increase Your Exposure to Daylight

You need to make sure that your body is being exposed to light during the day. Your body is going to recognize daylight as the time to be awake and the dark to be bedtime.

Making sure that you are exposed to light allows you to keep the regular rhythms of your sleep schedule. If you spend most of your day in a dark lit room it can be difficult to get your body on the right schedule.

Some of the ways that you can do this includes removing your sunglasses unless you are outside in really bright light. You should also spend more of your time outside when it is bright and sunny.

If you are stuck inside you should allow as much of the bright light into the area as you can by removing the blinds and the curtains and being as close to the window as you can.

When all else fails, you would be able to use a light therapy box which simulates the sunshine and can give you some benefits in the middle of winter when the sunlight is very limited.

Do as much as you can to get out in the light and sunshine in order to keep your sleep on track.

Health Tip #135 – How You Can Boost Melatonin Naturally at Night

Just as it is important to get the right amount of light during the day you will need to make sure that you are getting the melatonin production you need in order to fall asleep.

Some of the things that you can do in order to boost the melatonin that you are getting each night in order to fall asleep better include:

- Turning off the computer and television—there are many people who will use these two things in order to relax and fall asleep. But the light is going to make producing melatonin more difficult. These things can actually stimulate your mind instead of relaxing it so that it is more difficult to fall asleep.

- Never read from a device with a backlight—if you do use a device to read before bed, choose one that does not have a backlight and choose a lamp or other light source instead.

- Change out the bright bulbs—you want to have a lower light bulb in place to help tell your mind that it is night and time to go to bed.

- Keep your room dark—you should not go to sleep in a room that has a lot of lights. It is best if you are able to go to sleep in a room that is completely dark, but if you need a light for getting around or another reason, keep it low.

Health Tip #136 – Don't Sleep with Noises

You should make sure that your room is as quiet as possible for the best results. Keep the TV, radio, and other noises as low as possible.

Of course, you cannot control all of the noise such as traffic or barking dogs, you can make sure that you keep the noise down.

When there are other noises that are distracting you that cannot fall asleep, you should turn on some white noise.

Health Tip #137 – The Effect of Temperature When You Sleep

People will sleep much better if they are able to keep their bedroom at a temperature is that is a little bit cool.

You will find that it is more difficult to fall asleep in a room that is too warm and you might spend more time tossing and turning all around.

The best temperature to sleep at is about 65 degrees with some good ventilation. You should bring a blanket along to cover if you feel that this is too cold for you to handle.

Health Tip #138 – Bed Comfort is Compulsory

On your bed, you should make sure that there is enough room in order to turn around and stretch out comfortably.

You might want to try out a new mattress or even a new pillow if you find that you wake up with a sore neck or back.

Try some different firmness with the mattress; this does not mean that you have to buy a new mattress each time, but you can add some egg or foam crate toppers in order to get less or more support to get the best sleep.

You should also remember to keep the bed just for sex and for sleep. If you do other activities on the bed, it can confuse your mind and won't help to trigger that it is bedtime.

Health Tip #139 – Plan A Bedtime Ritual

You should make sure that you have a good bedtime ritual in place in order to start triggering your body to go to sleep.

Having this same ritual in place all of the time can make it easier to get the bed.

Some things that you can try out in order to have a good ritual would include things like:

- Taking a warm bath

- Reading a book or other material with a soft light

- Listening to some soft music

- Do stretches before bed

- Listen to a book on tape

- Find a simple hobby that will not get you too excited and do it in order to wind down.

These are just some of the things that you can do in order to fall asleep at night and wake up at a more natural time each day.

The sleep that you get is important to helping you to get the energy and recovery that you need so that the rest of your progress is not wasted.

Make sure that you are getting plenty of sleep each night for the best results.

I hope you have learned something from this book so far and would greatly appreciate it if you could leave an honest review on Amazon.com.

Discover Scientifically-Proven "Shortcuts" & "Hacks" to Lose Weight FASTER (With Very Little Effort)

For this month only, you can get Linda's best-selling & most popular book absolutely free – *Weight Loss Secrets You NEED to Know.*

Get Your FREE Copy Here:

TopFitnessAdvice.com/Bonus

Discover scientifically-proven tips to help you lose weight faster and easier than ever before. With this book, readers were able to improve their weight loss results and fitness levels. So, it's highly recommended that you get this book, especially while it's free!

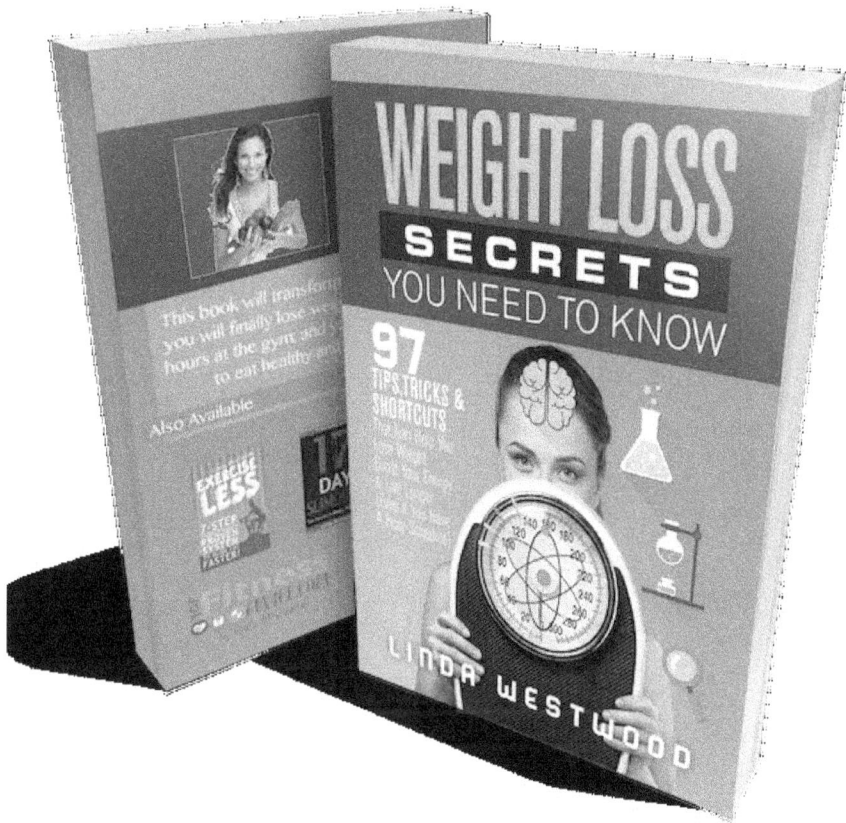

Get Your FREE Copy Here:

TopFitnessAdvice.com/Bonus

Conclusion

Use the tips in this book to make meaningful changes to your life that will help you get rid of the unwanted weight while toning and shaping your abs, butt, and thigh at the same time!

Remember to take your new weight loss plan one step at a time. If you try to make all the changes at once, you're likely to get burnt out.

It's better to make gradual changes so that you know they will stick and become permanent healthy habits.

Losing weight is about making these kinds of long-term lifestyle changes. That is the only way to burn off the fat *and* keep it off. So, put away this book and get moving!

Also, remember that your goal is to improve your overall health. Try to eat good food, sleep well, and take care of your body!

Final Words

I would like to thank you for purchasing my book and I hope I have been able to help you and educate you on something new.

If you have enjoyed this book and would like to share your positive thoughts, could you please take 30 seconds of your time to go back and give me a review on my Amazon book page.

I greatly appreciate seeing these reviews because it helps me share my hard work.

You can leave me a review on Amazon.com.

Again, thank you and I wish you all the best!

Enjoying this book?

Check out my other best sellers!

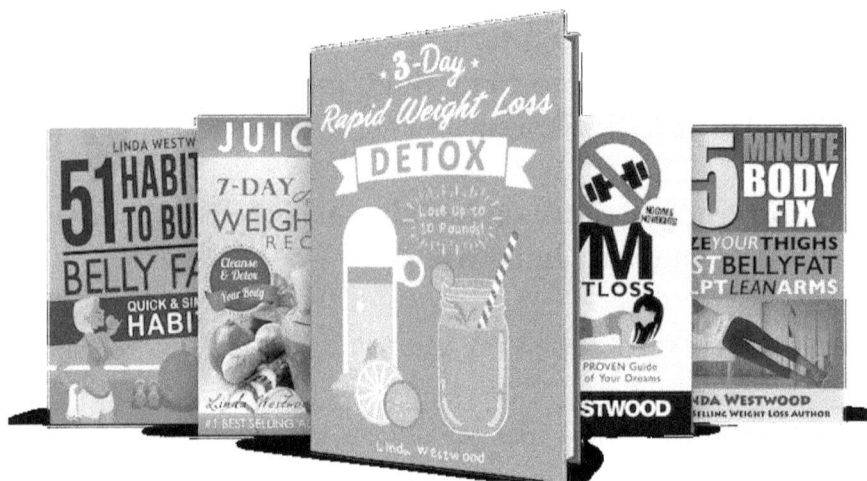

Get your next book on sale here:

TopFitnessAdvice.com/go/books